PALEO DIET FOR BEGINNERS

Home Cooking Made Easy With Paleo Cookbook!

(A Paleo Cookbook to Lose Weight and Reboot Your Health)

Victor Soper

Published by Alex Howard

Victor Soper

Paleo Diet for Beginners: Home Cooking Made Easy With Paleo Cookbook! (A Paleo Cookbook to Lose Weight and Reboot Your Health)

ISBN 978-1-77485-026-8

Legal & Disclaimer

The information contained in this book is not designed to replace or take the place of any form of medicine or professional medical advice. The information in this book has been provided for educational and entertainment purposes only.

The information contained in this book has been compiled from sources deemed reliable, and it is accurate to the best of the Author's knowledge; however, the Author cannot guarantee its accuracy and validity and cannot be held liable for any errors or omissions. Changes are periodically made to this book. You must consult your doctor or get professional medical advice before using any of the suggested remedies, techniques, or information in this book.

Upon using the information contained in this book, you agree to hold harmless the Author from and against any damages, costs, and expenses, including any legal fees potentially resulting from the application of any of the information provided by this guide. This disclaimer applies to any damages or injury caused by the use and application, whether directly or indirectly, of any advice or information presented, whether for breach of contract, tort, negligence, personal injury, criminal intent, or under any other cause of action.

You agree to accept all risks of using the information presented inside this book. You need to consult a professional medical practitioner in order to ensure you are both able and healthy enough to participate in this program.

Table of Contents

Part 1

Introduction

This book contains not just paleo recipes but also information that you need to know on what Paleo diet really is. It will help get rid of any doubts that you have in mind about paleo. This book also contains some misconceptions that you might have read in the internet. This will help you understand clearly why you shouldn't believe or believe people when they say that Paleo is an effective diet regimen.

If you are wondering what makes this book special and different from the rest, the book is written not to profit but to inform and educate people about paleo. For starters and who have been into paleo for a long time this is the perfect book for you. To help you out in preparing meals, the 99 recipes are categorized to breakfast, lunch, dinner, snacks, desserts and smoothies.

Thanks again for downloading this book, I hope you enjoy it!

Chapter 1: What You Can Get From Paleo Diet

If you haven't heard about paleo, then maybe you are not from earth. The paleo diet is one of the most popular and effective diet regimens these days. Some experts refer to this as the caveman diet. Paleo diet is considered as the healthiest way you can eat because it works with your genetics to help you stay strong, energized and lean. Research in biochemistry, dermatology, biology, biochemistry and other disciplines show that it is the modern diet, full of sugar, refined foods and trans fats that is at the root of degenerative diseases like diabetes, depression, obesity, infertility, heart disease and Parkinson's Alzheimer's.

The Principle

The paleo diet is similar to the food that hunter gathers: fruits, seafood, meats, nuts and vegetables. If you follow these nutritional guidelines, you can put your diet more in line with the evolutionary pressures that developed your genetics, which in turn affects the health and well-being positively. The paleo diet reduces the body's glycemic load, increases vitamin and nutrient consumption, balances carbohydrates, fat and proteins and has healthy ratio of unsaturated to saturated fatty acids.

The Paleo Diet

Fresh meat, fresh vegetables, and fresh fruits – the paleo diet is all about consuming foods on its natural state just like what the cavemen do. Experts suggest that if you want to eat healthy go for grass-fed and organic varieties if possible to limit your exposure to antibiotics, pesticides and other harmful chemicals.

Building a Paleo Diet

A. Lean Proteins

This will support healthy bones, immune function and strong muscles. The protein likewise makes you feel full between meals.

B. Fruits and Vegetables

The paleo diet includes fruits and vegetables that are rich in vitamins, phytonutrients, antioxidants, vitamins and minerals that have been proven that reduces the risk of having degenerative diseases like diabetes, neurological decline and cancer.

C. Healthy fats from Nuts, Seeds, Olive oil, Grass-fed Meat, Avocados, and Fish Oil

Based on Scientific Research and Epidemiological studies diet that is rich in Omega-3 fats and monounsaturated fats greatly reduce the possibilities of having cancer, heart disease, obesity, cognitive decline and diabetes.

Chapter 2: Misconceptions About Paleo Diet

As mentioned above the Paleo diet or Cave Man Diet focusses on eating the most natural state of the foods. There are some misconceptions circulating in the net about paleo diet and some of which are as follows:

1. The Paleo Diet is a Trend

Trend diets are shortsighted, mostly unhealthy regimens that promise immediate weight loss to profit from desperate dieters. Paleo diet is not a diet that will restrict you on the food you eat rather it is a lifestyle which main focus is optimal human nutrition. Some people apply paleo diet to help heal or treat serious health problems where traditional medicine was not able to provide. It is a grassroots movement, not a marketing strategy.

2. The Paleo Diet is basically a meat-eating diet.

Paleo diet is not at all a carnivorous diet. Most of the healthy paleo meals include seafood rather than red meat and usually get more calories from coconut products.

3. The Paleo Diet is Costly, Unsustainable and Limited.

Buying organic kale and grass-fed beef could be expensive but the price of medicines for diabetes and other diseases are more costly. The paleo diet may not be a reasonable option for everybody, but this is not the fault of the diet but of our present economic paradigm.

4. Restricting the whole food groups is unhealthy and restrictive.

Grains, legumes and dairy are not Paleo foods. Others think that cutting out the entire food groups may result to an unbalanced diet or deficiencies. However, dairy and grains only entered the human diet just recently, during the introduction of agriculture around 10,000 years ago. Definitely, there are no essential micronutrients, fatty acids or amino acids that can be found in grains, dairy or legumes.

5. The Paleo Diet is a Low-Carb Diet

Paleo does not restrict your carbohydrate intake especially if you are a highly active individual. If you cut out grains, legumes and their derivative and focuses on nutrient-dense whole foods, you will end up eating a lower amount of carbohydrate, thus you will feel less energized and may not be able to perform your daily activities properly.

6. The Paleo Diet works best only to men than women.

Although it is also known as the caveman diet, its effect is not only beneficial to men but to women as well. If you search online you will find out that the most influential champions of Paleo are actually women.

7. The Paleo diet is a one-size-fits-all approach.

There is no such thing as single approach for the Paleo diet. This diet should be seen as a template for a healthier lifestyle, drove by some fundamental nutritional principles but flexible in its approach.

Chapter 3: 20 Paleo Breakfast Recipes

Preparing a healthy breakfast for your family could be a daunting task especially if you are following a Paleo diet. Eggs are always an option, but sometimes you get tired of having it for breakfast. The good about paleo diet is that you are not asked to give up on muffins, waffles and pancakes. In this chapter you will find great tasting breakfast recipes that the whole family will truly love.

Paleo Almond-Cinnamon With Nutmeg Granola

INGREDIENTS:

1 ½ c. almond flour
2 teaspoon cinnamon
2 teaspoon nutmeg
2 teaspoon vanilla extract
½ c. walnuts
½ c. coconut flakes
¼ c. hemp hearts
Sea salt, to taste
1/3 c. coconut oil

DIRECTIONS:

•Pre-heat your oven to 275^{0}F.
•In a large mixing bowl place all the ingredients and mix well. To make sure the coconut oil will blend well with the other ingredients, you can melt it down first a little bit before adding.
•Grease a baking sheet and spread the mixture into one flat layer.
•Bake until the mixture is toasted depending on your preference or for 40 to 50 mins.

•Take it out of the oven and let it cool down before serving. Place the remaining granola into a plastic container.

NUTRITIONAL INFORMATION:

Calories   280
Fat   27.2g
Carbohydrates   6.4g
Fiber   3.3g
Protein   6.5g

Homemade Paleo Almond-Cinnamon Breakfast Bread

INGREDIENTS:

¼ tsp. baking soda
¼ tsp. celtic sea salt
¼ tsp. stevia
½ c. creamy roasted almond butter
1 tbsp. ground cinnamon
1 tsp. vanilla extract
2 large eggs
2 tbsp. honey

DIRECTIONS:

•Place the almond butter in a large bowl and mix using a hand blender until creamy.
•Add the honey, stevia, eggs and vanilla.
•Combine well using the blender until all the ingredients are added.
•Place the mixture into a greased 8 x 8 baking dish.
•Bake at 325 degree Fahrenheit for around 12 to 15 mins.
•Serve hot.

NUTRITIONAL INFORMATION:

Calories   270
Fat   21g
Carbohydrates   17g
Fiber   2g
Protein   8g
Sodium   270mg

Complete Paleo Breakfast Hash

INGREDIENTS:

1 1/2 teaspoon extra-virgin olive oil (or oil of choice)
1 cup chopped peppers and onions
1 finely chopped tomato
1 large chopped sweet potato
1 large handful fresh organic spinach
2 crushed garlic cloves
Himalayan sea salt and freshly ground pepper, to taste
Optional: 2 organic chopped chicken sausages
Optional: 4 pieces pre-cooked and chopped nitrate-free bacon

DIRECTIONS:

•Place a skillet over medium heat, add oil and saute garlic for 1 minute.
•Stir in sweet potato.
•After 4 to 5 mins. add in the onion, tomato and peppers.
•Saute for about 5 mins. with occasional stirring.
•Add in the bacon and sausage and let it cook for about 5 to 7 mins. with constant stirring.
•Add in the fresh spinach and continue cooking for another 2 to 3 mins. or until wilted.
•Transfer in a serving plate together with fresh organic eggs on top.

NUTRITIONAL INFORMATION:

Calories   290
Fat   19g
Carbohydrates   16g
Fiber   5g
Protein   14g
Sodium   860mg

Yummy Paleo Elvis Breakfast Cobbler

INGREDIENTS:

1 egg, beaten

1 piece cooked and crumbled center cut bacon

1/16 teaspoon baking soda (baking soda IS considered Paleo, while commercial baking powder is NOT.)

1/2 tablespoon pure maple syrup

1/8 teaspoon cinnamon

1/8 teaspoon pure vanilla extract

2 sliced bananas

2 tablespoons almond butter

2 tablespoons canned coconut milk

2 tablespoon coconut flour (ground-up coconut)

DIRECTIONS:

•Pre-heat your oven to 350^{0}F.

•Over medium heat place a small skillet coated with coconut oil. Add the bananas and let it cook for around 5 mins. flip when one side is brown.

•Combine baking soda, cinnamon and coconut flour in a small bowl.

•In another bowl combine coconut milk, vanilla, almond butter, maple syrup and egg. Whisk until well mixed.

•Add the almond butter mixture to coconut mixture and mix well. Add in the crumbled bacon. Pour the mixture over the bananas.

•Bake for 15 mins., or until a toothpick comes out clean when inserted into the dish.

NUTRITIONAL INFORMATION:

Calories	180
Fat	11g
Carbohydrates	18g
Fiber	2g

Protein   4g
Sodium   100mg

Hearty Avocado And Squash Paleo Breakfast

INGREDIENTS:

1 pound sugar-free sausage
1 sliced avocado
1/2 chopped red onion
2 cup shredded butternut squash,
2 tablespoon 100% Pure Avocado Oil
3 cup organic spinach
4 cloves minced garlic
4-6 eggs
4-6 slices chopped sugar-free grass-fed bacon
To garnish: chives or chopped scallions

DIRECTIONS:

•Heat a 12 inches cast iron skillet over medium heat and brown the bacon. Add the onion and avocado oil and cook until onion is translucent. Add the sausage and garlic. Cook for around 5 to 10 minutes or until the sausage becomes brown and crumbled.
•Set your broiler to high.
•Add the spinach and the shredded butternut squash and cook for 3 to 5 minutes more or until soft. Create small pockets in the mixture, enough to place the number of eggs you will be using. Carefully crack the eggs on each pockets, make sure that the yolks are intact.
•Broil until you achieve the desired done-ness. Broil longer if you prefer solid yolk, or if you want the yolk very runny broil it shorter.

NUTRITIONAL INFORMATION:

Calories   860
Fat   95g
Carbohydrates   24g
Fiber   8g
Protein   46g

Sodium   1600mg

Paleo Zucchini Pancake With Guacamole And Turkey On Top

INGREDIENTS:

For pancake
1 egg
1 zucchini, shredded
2 tablespoons almond flour
For the topping
2 eggs
1/2 cup fresh spinach
2 ounces turkey kielbasa
2 tbsp. guacamole
2 tbsp. diced jarred roasted red peppers

DIRECTIONS:

•Remove the water in zucchini by squeezing it.
•Combine the shredded zucchini with almond and egg flour. Add pepper and salt to taste.
•To form the mixture into 3 pancakes, use a non-stick skillet.
•Over a low heat cook the mixture for about 3 mins. on each side or until the inside cooks first before the outside burns. Set aside.
•Divide the spinach, turkey kielbasa and raw egg in small bowls or three 4 oz ramekins. Microwave until you achieve the desired doneness of the eggs or for about 1 minute.
•Place egg, kielbasa, spinach layer on top of each pancake and then add the diced red peppers and guacamole on top.

NUTRITIONAL INFORMATION:

Calories   190.50
Fat   12.4g
Carbohydrates   5.3g

Fiber	1.2g
Protein	14.6g
Sodium	573.7mg

Immune System Booster Paleo Breakfast Sausage

INGREDIENTS:

¼ tsp. cinnamon
¼ tsp. ginger
1 lb. ground pork
1 tbsp. maple syrup (optional)
1 tsp. dried rosemary
1 tsp. dried sage
1 tsp. salt

DIRECTIONS:

•Combine all the ingredients using your hands. To make the sausage taste better, allow it to sit in the fridge overnight before you cook it.
•Form into patties and fry over medium heat until slightly brown and cooked through or for about 3 to 5 minutes on each side.

NUTRITIONAL INFORMATION:

Calories   420
Fat   32g
Carbohydrates   5g
Fiber   0g
Protein   26g
    Sodium   870mg

Delicious Paleo Meatza Breakfast

INGREDIENTS:

1 pound bulk breakfast sausage
1 tsp minced garlic
1/2 diced small sweet potato
1/2 diced yellow onion
7 eggs
8 slices bacon, diced

DIRECTIONS:

•Pre-heat your oven to 350 degree Fahrenheit.
•Combine one egg and breakfast sausage by hand. Transfer in 8 x 8 pie or pan plate.
•Bake the mixture in oven for around 8 to 10 minutes. Remove excess fat.
•As you wait for the meat to cook, cook the bacon over medium heat until crispy.
•Place bacon in the paper towel to remove excess oil.
•Place 2 tablespoon of bacon oil in a pan and cook onion, garlic, and sweet potato for 8 to 10 minutes.
•Beat 6 eggs in a bowl.
•Arrange potato mixture on top of sausage.
•Pour the beaten eggs over the potato mixture.
•Sprinkle bacon bits on top of the eggs.
•Bake for about 8 to 10 minute or until the eggs are set.

NUTRITIONAL INFORMATION:

Calories   603.70
Fat   47.7g
Carbohydrates   5.5g
Fiber   0.7g
Protein   35.4g
Sodium   1117.2mg

Coconut Chai With Almonds Paleo Breakfast Bars

INGREDIENTS:

¼ c. honey
¼ teaspoon allspice
¼ teaspoon cloves
¼ teaspoon ground cardamom
⅓ c. coconut flour
½ c. sliced almonds, for topping
½ teaspoon cinnamon
½ teaspoon vanilla
¾ teaspoon powdered ginger
1 banana
1 c. unsweetened, shredded coconut
2 eggs
4 tablespoon coconut milk

DIRECTIONS:

•Pre-heat your oven to 350°F. Use coconut oil to grease an 8 x 8 inch baking pan.
•Whisk eggs in a medium size bowl.
•Add mashed banana into the eggs. Then add vanilla and honey.
•Sift the coconut flour, cinnamon, ginger, cardamom and cloves and the unsweetened shredded coconut.
•Mix well until there are no clumps, make sure the batter is thick enough and hold it's shape well.
•Spoon batter and place into greased pan. Spread evenly using a fork or spatula.
•Sprinkle almond on top of your bars in an even layer.
•Bake for 20 to 25 mins. or longer depending on the oven you use. The best way to check if the bars are done is to examine if it has little bits of golden brown coconut that is coming out through almonds on top. Use fork to test them if they are firm enough.

•You can store it in the fridge in the evening and serve it in the morning. To store them, score the bars while hot, and once they cool down, lift each square out of the pan and then place them into a freezer bag.

•The size of the bars is around 2.5 x 2.5 inches, it is hard to keep the bars shape if you cut them in bigger sizes.

•Before serving them, microwave them for about 30 seconds.

NUTRITIONAL INFORMATION:

Calories	150
Fat	8g
Carbohydrates	18g
Fiber	2g
Protein	3g
Sodium	45mg

Pumpkin Muffins With Almond-Apple Cider Caramel Streusel Toppings

INGREDIENTS:

¼ c. almond milk
¼ c. pumpkin puree
⅓ c. applesauce
½ c. coconut flour
½ c. coconut sugar or maple
½ c. tapioca flour
½ tbsp. Primal Palate Apple Pie Spice
½ tsp. baking powder
½ tsp. baking soda
1 apple, cored and diced
1 tsp. lemon juice
1 tsp. vanilla extract
3 eggs, whisked
    pinch of salt

For the streusel

1 tbsp. tapioca flour
2 tbsp. almond flour
2 tbsp. Tin Star Brown Butter
3 tbsp. maple sugar
Apple Cider Caramel

DIRECTIONS:

• Pre-heat your oven to 3500 Fahrenheit.
• In a big bowl, whisk together tapioca flour, apple pie spice, coconut flour, apple, baking soda and powder and salt. Add the rest of the ingredients and combine well.In forming the muffins use an ice cream scoop and place it in a silicone liner.
• In making the streusel, combine all the ingredients for the streusel in a small bowl. Add around ½ to 1 tsp. of the streusel on top of each muffin. Bake for about 30 mins. Meanwhile, make the apple cider caramel.
• Before removing the muffins from the silicone liner allow it to cool down a little bit. Place apple cider caramel on top of each muffin. Serve.

NUTRITIONAL INFORMATION:

Calories   120
Fat   3g
Carbohydrates   21g
Fiber   1g
Protein   3g
Sodium   190mg

Paleo Almond -Chocolate Zucchini Bread

INGREDIENTS:

1 3/4 c. finely grated zucchini
1 c. almond butter
1 tsp. vanilla extract
1/2 tsp. baking powder
1/2 tsp. baking soda
1/2 tsp. NuNaturals Liquid Vanilla Stevia
1/3 c. coconut sugar
1/4 c. coconut flour
1/4 c. unsweetened cocoa powder
1/4 tsp. sea salt
2 tsp. apple cider vinegar
5 large eggs, at room temperature

DIRECTIONS:

•Pre-heat your oven to 350⁰ Fahrenheit. Use parchment paper to line an 8.5 x 4.5 inches loaf pan and grease well.
•In a big mixing bowl, whisk together the eggs, vanilla extract, apple cider vinegar, vanilla stevia and almond butter until well combined.
•In another mixing bowl, sift together coconut flour, baking soda, coconut sugar, sea salt, unsweetened cocoa powder and baking powder.
•Add the dry ingredients into the wet ingredients and stir until well blended.
•Add the grated zucchini and combine well.
•Pour the mixture into the loaf pan, and bake until the toothpick comes out clean when poked into the center or for about 55-65 minutes.
•Remove the loaf from the pan and transfer on a cooling rack. Allow it to cool down completely before slicing.
NUTRITIONAL INFORMATION:

Calories	560
Fat	44g
Carbohydrates	31g
Fiber	5g
Protein	19g
Sodium	470mg

Paleo Waffle With Veggie Omelette And Bacon Toppings

INGREDIENTS:

For the waffles
¼ c unsweetened almond milk
¼ teaspoon baking soda
½ teaspoon gluten-free vanilla extract
1 tablespoon melted coconut oil
1/8 c coconut flour
2 eggs
Pinch of pumpkin pie spice
Pinch of salt

For the eggs
1 egg
1 slice uncured bacon
3 tablespoon liquid egg whites
Veggie fillings
drizzle of pure maple syrup
Salt and pepper to taste

DIRECTIONS:

In making the waffles:
•Pre-heat your waffle iron.
•In a medium bowl, combine all the ingredients, and whisk until well combined.
•Pour batter into the heated waffle iron and allow it to cook.

In making the eggs:
•While waiting for the waffles to cook, prepare the eggs.
•Heat a skillet over medium heat and add the olive oil.
•In a bowl combine liquid egg white, pepper, eggs and salt together. Put the egg mixture into the skillet. Then add the veggie or any toppings that you prefer.
•Slowly fold over to make an omelette. Set aside. On the same pan cook the bacon until the desired crispiness.

Assemble the meal:
•On top of one waffle place the omelette. Top it with bacon. You can add sliced avocado and drizzle some pure maple syrup on it. Do the same thing on the remaining waffle and serve.

NUTRITIONAL INFORMATION:

Calories   520
Fat   41g
Carbohydrates   15g
Fiber   5g
Protein   27g
Sodium   1900mg

Tilapia-Spinach Filled Paleo Burrito

INGREDIENTS:

For the tortillas
1/2 c. water
2 egg whites
2 eggs
4 teaspoon ground flaxseed
    Pinch of salt

For the filling
1 diced avocado
Handful of spinach leaves
1 teaspoon coconut oil
1/4 c. finely diced red bell pepper
1/4 c. finely diced onion
1/4 c. baked tilapia

DIRECTIONS:

•Whisk together all the ingredients for the tortilla in a small bowl. Pre-heat your oven broiler.
•Over medium fire, heat a ten inch nonstick skillet and coat with coconut oil spray.
•Pour ½ of the tortilla mixture in the pan and distribute evenly.
•Use a metal spatula to loosen the edges of the tortilla from the pan. Cook until golden brown on the bottom and then slowly slide the spatula under the tortilla. •Do not flip yet.
•Place the pan in the broiler for 3 to 4 minutes or until it becomes bubbly. •Remove the tortilla from the skillet, transfer it into a piece of aluminum foil. Do the same thing with the other half of tortilla mixture.
•Once you are done with your tortillas, pre-heat your oven to 400^0 Fahrenheit. •Over medium fire, heat another pan and add

the coconut oil. Add the peppers and onions and saute until soft or for about 5 to 8 mins. Place the spinach into the pan and wilt.
•Put the fillings in the center of the tortillas and tightly wrap. Place in the oven and cook for 5 to 8 mins. to set the shape of the tortilla. Serve.

NUTRITIONAL INFORMATION:

Calories	310
Fat	24g
Carbohydrates	15g
Fiber	9g
Protein	14g
Sodium	290mg

Baked Paleo Bacon With Avocado On Top

INGREDIENTS:

½ avocado
½ c. chopped tomatoes
2 Organic eggs
2 tablespoon chives
2 tablespoon pre-cooked crumbled bacon
Coconut oil
Salt and Pepper to taste

DIRECTIONS:

•Use coconut oil to grease a huge microwave safe bowl.
•Place the eggs in the bowl and microwave for around 1 minute.
•Add the chives, tomatoes and bacon and stir and then microwave again for 1 more minute.
•Place avocado on top. Add the salt and pepper to taste.
•Serve.

NUTRITIONAL INFORMATION:

Calories   110
Fat   8g
Carbohydrates   5g
Fiber   3g
Protein   6g
Sodium   320mg

Paleo Pumpkin-Chocolate Breakfast Bars with Shredded Coconut on Top

INGREDIENTS:

1 1/2 c. raw almonds
1 c. canned pumpkin
1 c. shredded unsweetened coconut
1 teaspoon pure vanilla extract
1/3 c. dark chocolate chips
1/4 teaspoon ground cinnamon
  2 tablespoon pure maple syrup

DIRECTIONS:

•Preheat oven to 350 degrees.
•Place almonds and coconut on a cooking sheet and place in oven for 15 minutes, or until slightly toasted.
•Add almonds and coconut to a food processor and process until it is a flour or meal-like texture. Add to a large bowl.
•In a small bowl combine pumpkin, maple syrup, vanilla and cinnamon. Add to almond-coconut mixture and mix well.
•Add in dark chocolate chips and use your hands to mix all ingredients together well.
•Spray cooking spray (or use parchment paper) in a large loaf pan and transfer the mixture to pan and use a spatula to smooth out. Sprinkle on shredded coconut.
•Bake for 25 minutes, or until golden brown.
•Let cool and slice into about 8 bars.

NUTRITIONAL INFORMATION:

Calories	460
Fat	33g
Carbohydrates	35g
Fiber	11g
Protein	13g

Sodium   65mg

Paleo Sweet Potato Noodles With Hollandaise Sauce

INGREDIENTS:

¼ tsp. garlic powder

1 diced avocado

1 large sweet potato, Blade C, noodles trimmed

1 tbsp. chopped cilantro

3 large eggs

Olive oil cooking spray

    Salt and pepper, to taste

    For the sauce:

½ tsp. sea salt

1 chipotle pepper + 1 tsp. of adobo sauce

1 tbsp. lemon juice

2 eggs yolks

3 tbsp. melted coconut oil

DIRECTIONS:

•Pre-heat your oven to 425⁰ Fahrenheit. Lightly coat with cooking spray a baking sheet, place the sweet potato noodle and season it with salt, pepper and garlic powder. Sprinkle avocado cubes on top and roast until the sweet potato noodles are cooked or for around 10 to 13 minutes.

•Meanwhile, place the lemon juice, sauce, egg yolks, chipotle pepper, and sea salt in a blender and pulse for around 10 seconds. Then, put the blender on medium and gradually add the coconut oil to thicken. Set aside.

•As soon as you are done with the hollandaise sauce, pour water in a medium saucepan fill it halfway and simmer.

•Break the eggs into a small bowl or ramekin. Then, make a gentle whirlpool in the simmering water so the egg white will wrap around the yolk. Gradually tip the egg into the water. Cook for 3 mins. Take the eggs out of the water using a slotted spoon and transfer it on a paper towel lined plate.

•As soon as the avocado and sweet potato noodles are done, make a nest on 3 plates. Place poached eggs on top and drizzle with hollandaise sauce.

•Serve and garnish it with cilantro.

NUTRITIONAL INFORMATION:

Calories	400
Fat	33g
Carbohydrates	20g
Fiber	8g
Protein	11g
Sodium	1100mg

Paleo Sweet Potato Beef Burger With Avocado And Bacon Recipe

INGREDIENTS:

¼ pound bacon
¼ teaspoon black pepper
½ chopped onion
½ head romaine lettuce
½ tablespoon lime juice
½ teaspoon salt
1 avocado
1 large sweet potato
1 pound ground beef
1 sliced red bell pepper
1 tablespoon olive oil or fat of choice
2 minced garlic cloves

DIRECTIONS:

•Pre-heat your oven to 400 degrees Fahrenheit.
•Rinse the sweet potato and slice into ½ inch.
•Use parchment paper or foil to line two baking sheets, coat with olive oil and arrange the sweet potato slices on it. On the other sheet lay the bacon.
•Bake the bacon and sweet potato slices for around 20 to 25 mins. Flip halfway through. Meanwhile, prepare the bell pepper, onions and burgers, and smash the avocado.
•Combine minced garlic, pepper, ground beef, and salt and form into 6 patties.
•In a large skillet heat olive oil over medium heat and cook the patties for around 5 mins. on each side.
•In another skillet heat olive oil over medium heat and cook the onions and bell pepper until slightly charred and soft.
•Smash the lime juice and avocado in a medium bowl. Add pepper and salt to taste.

•Arrange each slider by putting sweet potato slice with lettuce on top, burger patty, smashed avocado, onions, bacon and bell pepper and another slice of sweet potato.

NUTRITIONAL INFORMATION:

Calories	370
Fat	28g
Carbohydrates	12g
Fiber	5g
Protein	19g
Sodium	420mg

Paleo Maple Glazed Cinnamon-Banana With Walnut Donuts

INGREDIENTS:

2 beaten eggs
1/2 teaspoon baking soda
1/2 teaspoon cinnamon
1 1/2 mashed ripe bananas
1/2 teaspoon vanilla extract
1 1/2 tablespoon maple syrup
1/2 c. chopped walnuts
1/4 c. coconut flour
1/8 teaspoon ground cloves
1/8 teaspoon nutmeg

Glaze
3 tablespoon maple syrup
1 tablespoon melted coconut oil

DIRECTIONS:

• Pre-heat your oven to 350 degrees Fahrenheit.
• In a large bowl combine baking soda, cinnamon, flour, cloves and nutmeg. Combine well.
• In another bowl, combine maple syrup, banana, vanilla and eggs. Combine well and add to flour mixture.
• Add the walnuts and stir until evenly combined.
• Spray in a donut tin the cooking spray and place the batter. Bake until done or for around 20 minutes.
• Allow it to cool down and remove it from the donut pan.
• Serve.

NUTRITIONAL INFORMATION:

Calories   180

Fat   11g
Carbohydrates   19g
Fiber   2g
Protein   4g
Sodium   130mg

Baked Paleo Carrot With White Choco Chips Breakfast Cake

INGREDIENTS:

6 tablespoon coconut flour
2 tablespoon apple sauce
1 egg, beaten (or flax egg)
6 tablespoon almond milk
1 teaspoon vanilla
2 tablespoon raisins
1 tablespoon paleo friendly white chocolate chips
1 tablespoon crushed walnuts
1/2 teaspoon baking powder
1/2 tablespoon maple syrup
1/4 c. grated carrot

DIRECTIONS:

•Pre-heat your oven to 350 degrees Fahrenheit.
•Combine baking powder and coconut flour in a bowl.
•Add the other ingredients and stir until all ingredients are well combined.
•In a small cast iron skillet spray cooking spray and add spoonful of mixture and spread evenly.
•Bake until done or for around 35 minutes.
•Serve.

NUTRITIONAL INFORMATION:

Calories   80
Fat   4g
Carbohydrates   9g
Fiber   1g
Protein   3g
Sodium   105mg

Tasty Paleo Egg Muffins

INGREDIENTS:

4 organic eggs
1 tomato
Salt & Pepper to taste
1/2 onion
1/3 c. of nitrate free, organic bacon

DIRECTIONS:

•Preheat your oven to 18⁰C.
•Slice meat, tomato and onion and place on the pan and cook. Season.
•Place into silicon muffin liners, fill them up ¼ to 1/3 way up.
•Whisk four eggs and add into muffin liners around ¾ full.
•Bake for 15 mins. and serve with tomato, carrot batons and fresh avocado.

NUTRITIONAL INFORMATION:

Calories   200
Fat   15g
Carbohydrates   6g
Fiber   2g
Protein   12g
Sodium   510mg

Chapter 4: 20 Paleo Lunch Recipes

Serving the right meal for lunch is such a challenge particularly for paleo lovers. If you are following the paleo meal plan, you need to serve meal that contains meat, nuts, fish and seafood, veggies, fruits, tubers, healthy fats and oils and eggs. The following recipes are easy to prepare and flavorful meal that will keep you focused and awake for the entire day.

Healthy Spicy Avocado Stuffed With Tuna And Pepper

INGREDIENTS:

1 c. roughly chopped cilantro leaves
1 diced red bell pepper
1 lime, juiced
1 minced jalapeno
3 (4.5 oz) cans tuna, drained
4 halved and pitted avocados
Salt and pepper

DIRECTIONS:

•Create a bowl like space at the center of the avocado by scooping out some of its flesh.
•Place the scooped part into a medium size bowl and mash it using a fork.
•Add bell pepper, cilantro, tuna and jalapeno to the mashed avocado. Add lime juice and stir until well combined.
•Scoop the tuna mixture and place it in the avocado bowls.
•Season with pepper and salt to taste. Serve.

NUTRITIONAL INFORMATION:

Calories   320
Fat   23g

Carbohydrates   17g
Fiber   11g
Protein   18g
Sodium   170mg

Paleo Veggie Sandwich Rounds

INGREDIENTS:
1/4 cup coconut flour
1/4 cup milk of choice or water
2 eggs
2 smallish-medium-sized carrots
Salt and pepper, to taste
Optional: Real Salt Seasoning Salt or 1/2 tsp. Herbes de Provence or Herbamare

DIRECTIONS:

•Pre-heat your oven to 400^0F and use parchment paper to line a baking sheet or a silpat mat.
•Place coconut and carrots in your food processor and pulse until the mixture looks like orange crumbs or for about 30 to 60 secs. add the remaining ingredients into the food processor and process until smooth or for 1 min.
•Divide into eight parts and form into rounds on the baking sheet. Flatten the rounds with your hands. Dampen your hands to prevent it from sticking to your hands. The patties should be around ¼ inch thick, not too think for it will not hold together.
•Bake until slightly brown on the bottom or for about 15 to 17 minutes and dry on the top.
•Allow it to cool down for a few minutes before taking it out of the pan. Serve within an hour of baking.
•You can prepare extra and place it in a freezer-safe bag and store it in the freezer.

NUTRITIONAL INFORMATION:

Calories   35
Fat   1.5g
Carbohydrates   3g
Fiber   1g
Protein   2g
Sodium   135mg

Paleo Almond-Coconut with Flaxseed Sandwich Bread

INGREDIENTS:

1 tablespoon honey
1 teaspoon apple cider vinegar
1 teaspoon baking soda
1/2 teaspoon salt
1/4 c. ground flaxseed meal
1/4 c. melted coconut oil
3 tablespoon coconut flour
3/4 c. almond butter
5 eggs

DIRECTIONS:

•Pre-heat your oven to 3500 Fahrenheit. Use parchment paper to line a loaf pan.
•In a big bowl combine eggs, honey, apple cider vinegar, coconut oil, and almond butter use a hand blender to mix them together.
•In another bowl, combine coconut flour, salt, baking soda, and flaxseed meal. •Add the dry ingredients into the wet ingredients.
•Place the dough into the baking pan. Bake for 30 to 35 minutes until completely set and brown.
•Take it out of the oven and let the loaf cool down in the pan for ten minutes, then remove it from the pan and place on a wire rack to allow it to cool down completely.
•Store in an airtight container and refrigerate.

NUTRITIONAL INFORMATION:

Calories   520
Fat   47g
Carbohydrates   15g
Fiber   2g

Protein   15g
Sodium   700mg

Paleo Bok Choy Stir-Fry Burger

INGREDIENTS:

1 tbsp. soy sauce or 1 tbsp. coconut aminos

1 tsp. chili powder

1 tsp. freshly grated ginger

2 diced bell peppers

2 eggs

2 hamburger patties precooked diced or 1⁄2 lb minced meat

2 tsp. red chili pepper flakes

3 tbsp. coconut oil, divided

6 bunches washed bok choy

Salt & freshly ground black pepper, to taste

   Salt, to taste

DIRECTIONS:

•Place one tablespoon of coconut oil in a pan and heat over medium heat. Add bell peppers and meat and stir fry until the bell peppers are cooked.

•Add red pepper flakes, salt, pepper, soy sauce, and chili powder.

•Remove the ends of the bok choy and pull the leaves apart.

•Heat the pan and add again and add one tablespoon coconut oil and stir fry bok choy leaves until wilted. Add the salt and grated ginger.

•Fry eggs depending on your preferred doneness.

•Divide the stir-fried bell peppers into two bowls. Place the bok chow leaves on the side of the bowl. Place the fried egg on top.

NUTRITIONAL INFORMATION:

Calories	836.2
Fat	44g
Carbohydrates	64g
Fiber	28.8g
Protein	70.2g
Sodium	2357.6mg

Mashed Avocado With Bacon Toppings In Lettuce Wrap

INGREDIENTS:

1 ripe avocado
1/2 teaspoon lemon juice
1/4 teaspoon mustard (omit for AIP)
1/4 teaspoon sea salt
2 strips cooked bacon
3-4 leaves butter lettuce
4 ounce can wild tuna or chicken
Garlic powder
Onion powder
Parsley flakes

DIRECTIONS:

•Slice the avocado and mash it in a bowl and add chicken or tuna.
•Season with garlic powder, parsley, onion powder, lemon juice and mustard.
•Rip off lettuce leaves and add a spoonful of avocado mixture in each leaf.
•Slice the bacon to preferred size and add it to the leaf.
•Eat using your hands and enjoy.

NUTRITIONAL INFORMATION:

Calories   140
Fat   10g
Carbohydrates   7g
Fiber   4g
Protein   8g
Sodium   210mg

Scorched Tuna Nicoise Veggie Salad Recipe

INGREDIENTS:

1 tbsp. extra-virgin olive oil

1 tbsp. fresh lemon juice

1 tsp. Dijon mustard

1 tsp. water

1/2 c. halved cherry tomatoes

1/2 minced garlic clove

1/4 c. fresh basil leaves

1/4 thinly sliced red onion

1/4 tsp. kosher salt

1/4 tsp. maple syrup

2 c. petite lettuce leaves

2 cooled and sliced hard-boiled eggs

2 mini cucumbers, sliced thin crosswise

2 oz. French green beans, trimmed

2 tsp. capers

4 thinly sliced radishes

8-oz. tuna steak

Fresh cracked black pepper

Olive oil cooking spray

DIRECTIONS:

•Boil water in a medium size bowl. Add the beans and cook for around 2 mins. or until crisp-tender and bright green. Remove the water and add ice water on it. •Drain and then set aside.
•Divide and arrange basil, cucumbers, eggs, lettuce, radishes, green beans, tomatoes, and onion evenly between 2 plates.
•Over medium-high heat, heat a large nonstick skillet. Use cooking spray to coat the pan.
•Sprinkle tuna with pepper and salt.
•Add the tuna into the pan and cook for about 2 mins. on each side or until brown on the outside but pink inside.
•Cut thinly across the grain. Place tuna on top of the veggies.
•In preparing the dressing, combine lemon juice and the remaining ingredients in a small jar and cover it tightly. Shake well and drizzle over salads evenly.

NUTRITIONAL INFORMATION:

Calories   350
Fat   17g
Carbohydrates   10g
Fiber   3g
Protein   38g
Sodium   523mg

Paleo Bacon And Egg Salad Recipe

INGREDIENTS:

12 hard-boiled eggs
1 medium red onion
Nom Nom Paleo's Mayo
6-7 pieces crumbled bacon
Optional: sliced almonds, grapes, raisins

DIRECTIONS:

•Fry the bacon depending on your preferred doneness.
•Hard boiled the eggs and chop the onions into small pieces.
•Combine all the ingredients together in a bowl. The mayo will serve as a binder.
•Store in the fridge and serve it cold.

NUTRITIONAL INFORMATION:

Calories   370
Fat   26g
Carbohydrates   12g
Fiber   1g
Protein   22g
Sodium   340mg

Paleo Curried Chicken Salad

INGREDIENTS:

¼ c. chopped onions
¼ c. fresh chopped dill
¼ c. slivered almonds
¼ teaspoon turmeric
½ c. chopped apples
½ c. mayo
½ lime, juiced
½ teaspoon sea salt
¾ teaspoon curry powder
2 cooked chicken breasts, cut into small chunks
Fresh ground pepper

DIRECTIONS:

•Combine the curry, pepper, dill, turmeric and salt in a small bowl. Put aside.
•Stir together the chopped apples with the fresh lime juice in a medium bowl.
•Add the onions and chicken and stir again. Add in the dressing and coat well the apples and chicken.
•Serve on top of greens with slivered almonds.

NUTRITIONAL INFORMATION:

Calories   180
Fat   13g
Carbohydrates   15g
Fiber   3g
Protein   2g
Sodium   510mg

Roasted Paleo Butternut Squash Soup

INGREDIENTS:

1 1/2 teaspoon salt
1 large butternut squash
1 sliced and cored green apple
1 small chopped yellow onion
1 teaspoon chili powder
1/2 teaspoon cumin
2 chopped carrots
2 tablespoon ghee
2 teaspoon cinnamon
3 cups chicken broth
    3 tablespoon olive oil

DIRECTIONS:

•Pre-heat your oven to 400^{0} Fahrenheit. In a big bowl, combine 1 teaspoon cinnamon, butternut squash, ½ teaspoon cumin, olive oil, and ½ teaspoon salt. •Combine together, coat the squash well. On a rimmed baking sheet spread out the mixture.

•Toss the onion, carrots, apple slices in a bowl with butternut squash to coat with the remnants.

•Place the mixture on a second rim baking sheet and place both the baking sheets in the oven. Roast for 35 to 40 mins. until soft, stir once.

•In a large pot heat up ghee over medium heat, add the roasted ingredients and then pour the chicken broth.

•Add 1 tsp. of each cinnamon, chili powder and salt. Boil and then lower the heat to simmer, cover for 20 mins.

•Use an immersion blender, put the ingredients until smooth, or place in a blender to puree.

•Serve warm.

NUTRITIONAL INFORMATION:

Calories   220
Fat   10g
Carbohydrates   29g
Fiber   4g
Protein   3g
Sodium   610mg

Paleo Chicken And Veggies Tortilla Soup Recipe

INGREDIENTS:

1 28ounce can of diced tomatoes
1 bunch chopped fine of cilantro
1 diced sweet onion
1 teaspoon chili powder
1 teaspoon cumin
1-2 c. water
2 c. chopped celery
2 c. of shredded carrots
2 de-seeded and diced jalepenos
2 large skinless chicken breasts, cut into ½ inch strips
2 tablespoon tomato paste
32 oz. organic chicken broth
4 cloves minced garlic
Olive oil
Sea salt & fresh cracked pepper to taste

DIRECTIONS:

•Heat a large dutch oven or crockpot over medium high heat, add a dash of olive oil and ¼ cup of chicken broth.
•Add garlic, sea salt, pepper, jalapeno and onions and cook until soft, add more broth as needed.
•Add all the remaining ingredients and water to fill the pot. Cover and cook for 2 hours on low and add pepper and salt to taste if needed.
•Shred the cooked chicken using the back of a wooden spoon and pressing it at the side of the pot. You can also use a tongs or fork to break the chicken apart and shreds it.
•Top with fresh cilantro and avocado slices. Serve.

NUTRITIONAL INFORMATION:

Calories   230
Fat   7.5g
Carbohydrates   8.3g
Fiber   1.8g
Protein   31.6g
Sodium   822mg

Paleo Baked Yams With Sloppy Joes Mixture Recipe

INGREDIENTS:

4 pre-baked yams
1 clove minced garlic
1 tablespoon of chili powder
1 teaspoon of cumin
2 tablespoon of coconut sugar or honey
(1) 14 ounce can of diced tomatoes, with liquids
(1) 6 ounce can of tomato paste
1 1/2 pounds of grass-fed ground beef
1/2 small chopped onion
1/2 chopped green pepper
1/2 chopped red pepper, small
1/4 c. chopped celery, small

DIRECTIONS:

•Saute the garlic, onions and celery in a skillet until the onions become tender.
•Add the ground beef and cook in the same skillet.
•Add the coconut sugar, bell peppers and spices to the skillet.
•Add the diced tomatoes with the liquid and the tomato paste.
•Simmer on low for around 15 mins.
•Add pepper and salt to taste.
•Slice sweet potatoes in half and form a little bowl in the center and fill it with the mixture.
•Serve warm and enjoy.

NUTRITIONAL INFORMATION:

Calories   570
Fat   26g
Carbohydrates   47g
Fiber   8g

Protein   39g
Sodium   550mg

Tasty Paleo Roasted Shrimp Cocktail

INGREDIENTS:

1 lb. uncooked shrimp, peeled, deveined, and thawed if frozen
1 tbsp. olive oil
Lemon wedges
Paleo cocktail sauce
sea salt and fresh ground pepper to taste

DIRECTIONS:

•Pre-heat your oven to 425 degrees Fahrenheit.
•Toss shrimp with oil, pepper and salt and place it on rimmed baking sheet in single layer.
•Roast and turn once for around 5 to 10 minutes depending on how big the shrimp or until the shrimp is pink and cooked through.
•Serve chilled with lemon wedges and paleo cocktail sauce.

NUTRITIONAL INFORMATION:

Calories   20
Fat   0.18g
Carbohydrates   1.67g
Fiber   0.5g
Protein   2.51g
Sodium   182mg

Protein Rich Paleo Pork With Lemon And Tomato

INGREDIENTS:

½ teaspoon cayenne pepper
½ teaspoon paprika
1 6ounce - 8ounce can organic tomato paste
1 chopped onion
1 seeded jalapeno pepper
1 teaspoon cumin
1 teaspoon thyme
2 pounds pork loin
2 tablespoon lemon juice
2 teaspoon chili powder
3 tablespoon coconut oil
4 minced garlic cloves

DIRECTIONS:

•Put all the ingredients in a crock pot.
•Set the crock pot on low and cook for five hours
•Shred the pork using two forks.
•Serve warm.

NUTRITIONAL INFORMATION:

Calories   382
Fat   17g
Carbohydrates   18g
Fiber   0g
Protein   40g
Sodium   138mg

Paleo Chicken Curry With Green Beans Recipe

INGREDIENTS:

1 cup tomatoes
1 tablespoon olive oil
1 teaspoon cayenne pepper
1 teaspoon salt
2 cups cooked chicken
2 tablespoon butter
2 teaspoon pepper
280 g onion
3 cups chicken stock
3 diced hot peppers
4 tablespoon curry powder
5 clove garlic
8 oz. green beans

DIRECTIONS:

•Heat olive oil and saute garlic, pepper and onion.
•Add diced chicken and cook for 5 mins.
•Add spices and stir.
•Add crushed tomatoes and chicken stock and stir well.
•Add in butter and stir.
•Cook for about 20 mins.
•Adjust salt and pepper to taste.
•Add green beans and stir and continue cooking for another 10 mins.
•Let it stand for 10 minutes before serving.
•Serve on top of cauliflower couscous.

NUTRITIONAL INFORMATION:

Calories   193
Fat   8.7g

Carbohydrates   14.3g
Fiber   4.4g
Protein   16.6g
Sodium   837mg

Nutritious Chipotle Chicken In Lettuce Wraps

INGREDIENTS:

Splash of olive oil (for frying)
1 400g tin of tomatoes
400g of skinless chicken breast cut into thin strips
1 finely sliced red onion
1 tablespoon of finely chopped chipotle in adobo sauce
Salt and pepper to season
1/2 teaspoon cumin
Lettuce leaves to make your tacos
Fresh coriander leaves
Slices of avocado
Pinch of brown sugar
Sliced pickled jalapeno
Lime wedges to spritz

Rustic salsa:

Cherry tomatoes
Sliced red onions
Scallions
Salt and pepper to taste

DIRECTIONS:

•Heat a nonstick frying pan over medium heat and add the olive oil. Fry chicken pieces until golden brown. Put aside.
•Add more olive oil in the same pan and fry onion until softens.
•Add cumin, chipotle, tomatoes and cumin and simmer for around 15 to 25 mins. until the tomato sauce thickens on the pan edges.
•Add the chicken back in the sauce and cook for 5 mins.
•Arrange the ingredients to make your tacos in another bowl and serve. You can sprinkle lime juice to improve the flavor.

NUTRITIONAL INFORMATION:

Calories   515
Fat   17.5g
Carbohydrates   49g
Fiber   8g
Protein   46.5g
Sodium   1135mg

Paleo Lettuce Wraps With Picadillo Fillings

INGREDIENTS:

For the Picadillo
¼ c. currants
½ tsp. ground cinnamon
½ tsp. salt
1 14 ounce can whole tomatoes
1 large green bell pepper, about 1.5 cups diced
1 lb. ground beef, (grass-fed)
1 medium onion, about 1.5 cups diced small
1 tsp. freshly ground black pepper
1 tsp. ground cumin
2 tbsp. drained capers
2 tbsp. green olives with pimiento, diced
2 tbsp. olive brine
2 tbsp. tallow, lard, or coconut oil

For the Pico de Gallo
⅓ c. minced shallot or red onion
⅔ c. diced tomatoes
2 tbsp. minced cilantro
2 tsp. fresh lime juice
Salt to taste

To Serve
Chopped cilantro (optional)
Cooked brown or white rice (optional)
Lettuce leaves or cabbage leaves

DIRECTIONS:

•Over medium heat, heat a Dutch oven or large skillet. Add the beef. Stir and crumble. Once cooked remove from heat and put aside.
•Add oil in the pan. Saute onions and cook until it starts to soften, or for around 3 to 4 mins.
•Add the bell pepper and cook for 3 minutes more.

•Add the garlic, black pepper, cinnamon, salt, and cumin and stir for 30 secs. until fragrant.

•Add the cooked beef, currants, capers, canned tomatoes, olive brine and diced olives. Break the tomatoes into small pieces as the mixture boil.

•Lower the heat to low, place the lid and simmer for 10 to 20 minutes.

•Prepare the pico de gallo while waiting. Combine chopped tomatoes, lime juice, shallot, cilantro and a dash of salt, then put aside.

•Place beef mixture on lettuce leaf, a spoonful of pico de gallo and a spoonful of rice if you want. Enjoy.

NUTRITIONAL INFORMATION:

Calories   246
Fat   10.8g
Carbohydrates   17.9g
Fiber   0g
Protein   17.9g
Sodium   590mg

Healthy Chicken Shawarma With Lemon-Basil Vinaigrette

INGREDIENTS:

Chicken Shawarma
1 lb / organic chicken breast, cut into 3-inch strips
2 tbsp. olive oil
2 tbsp. lemon juice
¾ tsp. fine grain sea salt
3 minced garlic cloves
1 tsp. curry powder
½ tsp. ground cumin
¼ tsp. ground coriander
Salad
6 cups spring greens
1 cup cherry tomatoes, halved
2 handfuls torn fresh basil leaves
1 sliced avocado
Lemon-Basil Vinaigrette
2 large handfuls fresh basil leaves
1 clove smashed garlic
½ tsp. fine grain sea salt
2 tbsp. fresh lemon juice
5 tbsp. olive oil

DIRECTIONS:

•Whisk lemon juice, curry powder, coriander, garlic, cumin, olive oil and cumin until well mixed.
•In a large Ziploc bag or sealable container combine chicken strips and marinade.
•Seal and marinate the chicken for at least 20 mins. in the fridge or you can marinate it overnight.
•When it is time to cook the meal, heat a big nonstick skillet over med-high heat.
•Add a small amount of olive oil, then add the chicken and cook until golden brown or for about 6 to 8 mins. turn regularly, until the juice run clear.
•Meanwhile, prepare the vinaigrette. Add the basil, salt, lemon juice, basil, salt and garlic in the blender until smooth. Slowly add the oil while the blender is still running. Process until well mixed. Put aside.
•In preparing the salads, add the greens in a huge bowl and toss, sprinkle pepper and salt. Add the chicken on top together with basil, avocado and tomatoes.
•Drizzle lemon-basil vinaigrette.
•Serve.

NUTRITIONAL INFORMATION:

Calories   392
Fat   28g
Carbohydrates   9g
Fiber   0g
Protein   27g

Spicy Paleo Pork And Pepper Stew

INGREDIENTS:

½ c. fresh chopped basil
½ tsp. cumin seed, whole
1 medium diced onion
1 medium lime, juiced
1 medium red bell pepper, seeded and diced
1 medium yellow bell pepper, seeded and diced
1 tsp. chili powder
1/8 tsp. freshly ground black pepper, to taste
1/8 tsp. sea salt, to taste
2 lbs. pork shoulder roast, cut into chunks
2 medium jalapeno pepper, seeded and diced
2 tbsp. olive oil
3 medium garlic cloves, minced
3 tbsp. tomato paste
4 c. chicken broth

DIRECTIONS:

•Over medium high heat, heat the olive oil. Add the meat and cook until cooked through and brown on all sides. Remove the pork from the pan using a slotted spoon and put aside.
•Add onions and peppers and cook until soft. Add chili powder, garlic and cumin and cook for 1 min. add the meat back to the pan.
•Add the tomato paste and chicken broth. Let it boil and then simmer until the meat is tender or for about 2 hours.
•Use two forks to shred the pork and add in the lime juice. Season to taste and serve warm.

NUTRITIONAL INFORMATION:

Calories   408

Fat   23.7g
Carbohydrates   14.8g
Protein   34.2g
Sodium   737mg

Protein-Rich Pork Tenderloin With Cilantro And Lime Tacos

INGREDIENTS:

1 1/2 c. thinly sliced onion
1 lb. pork tenderloin, trimmed and cut into thin strips
1 small seeded and chopped jalapeño pepper
1/2 c. chopped plum tomato
1/2 c. fat-free, less-sodium chicken broth
1/4 tsp. salt
1/8 tsp. freshly ground black pepper
2 1/2 tbsp. fresh lime juice
2 tsp. olive oil
3 tbsp. chopped cilantro
8 (6-inch) flour tortillas

DIRECTIONS:

•Over med-high fire, heat a large non-stick skillet. Add oil to the pan and saute pork with salt and black pepper for 4 minutes or until golden brown.
•Take it out of the pan and place it in a bowl.
•Add jalapeno and onion to the pan and saute for 5 mins. or until tender.
•Add the broth, lower the heat and simmer for 1 min. scrape pan to remove the browned bits. Add in tomato and simmer for 2 mins.
•Return the pork and the juices to the pan. Add lemon juice and cilantro and cook for 1 min. or until the meat is cooked through.
•Heat the tortillas as indicated in the package. Add ½ cup pork mixture in each tortilla and roll up.

NUTRITIONAL INFORMATION:

Calories   416
Fat   13.1g

Carbohydrates   43.1g
Protein   30.2g
Sodium   569mg

INGREDIENTS:

1 (28 ounce) can fired-roasted, crushed tomatoes
1 head cauliflower (florets only)
1 pound ground, seasoned sausage
1/2 teaspoon granulated garlic
1/2 teaspoon red pepper flakes (optional)
2 tablespoon butter
2 tablespoon Italian seasoning
2 teaspoon sea salt (or to taste)
3 medium chopped leeks (whites and light green sections)
    Juice of 1/2 lemon

DIRECTIONS:

•Over med-high heat, heat a 3 to 4 quart pan. Add leeks and butter and saute for 3 to 5 mins.

•Add sausage and cook with frequent stirring until the meat is cooked through.

•Add Italian seasoning, lemon, tomatoes, granulated garlic and red pepper flakes. •Simmer over medium heat for 20 mins. and stir occasionally.

•While waiting, microwave the cauliflower for 5 mins. and process in a food processor until you achieve the desired consistency.

•Add sea salt to season the tomato sauce and sausage and serve over the cauliflower.

NUTRITIONAL INFORMATION:

Calories   558
Fat   32g
Carbohydrates   28g
    Protein   27g

Chapter 5: 20 Paleo Dinner Recipes

If you are following a paleo diet, you should use grass fed and pastured meat, wild-caught seafood and fresh veggies. Seeds and fruit nuts should be used in moderation. Nutritionists, physicians and other researchers are recommending this type of diet not just for those who want to lose weight but also for those who want to stay healthy and maintain their body. Also there is some evidence that people who eat this way reduce their risk of getting sick. The following paleo dinner recipes are easy to follow and contain good amount of protein, sodium, fiber that is low in fat and calories.

Three Spices Paleo Chicken Strips Recipe

INGREDIENTS:
1 tablespoon Basil
1 tablespoon Oregano
1 tablespoon Thyme
3 Cups Coconut flour
    3 Organic Eggs

DIRECTIONS:
• Slice the chicken into one inch strips to produce around 21 strips and 5 inches long.
• Separate egg whites and egg yolk.
• Place the egg whites in a bowl and beat add 2 tablespoon of water.
• Toss chicken in the white eggs and make sure they are covered.
• Pre-heat your oven to 400 degrees Fahrenheit.
• In a medium size mixing bowl combine basil, thyme, oregano and coconut flour.
• Add the coated chicken into the spice mixture and cover completely.

•Arrange the chicken fingers on a parchment paper.
•Bake for 10 to 12 minutes then flip over.
•Bake for another 8 to 12 minutes or until golden brown.
•Take it out of the oven and allow it to cool down for 5 minutes.
•Serve.

NUTRITIONAL INFORMATION:
Calories   10
Fat   0.5g
Carbohydrates   0g
Protein   1g
Sodium   10mg

Healthy Paleo Mexican Casserole

INGREDIENTS:

1 dice red bell pepper
1 pound Chorizo
1 teaspoon Salt
1/2 teaspoon Pepper
12 Eggs
1 tablespoon avocado oil
4-5 thinly sliced Green onions/Scallions
Cilantro to garnish

DIRECTIONS:

• Pre-heat your oven to 375 degrees Fahrenheit.
• Brown the chorizo and drain.
• Spread avocado oil in a casserole dish.
• Place the chorizo at the bottom of the casserole dish.
• Thinly slice the green onions and dice the red bell pepper.
• Break eggs in a big bowl and whisk to mix well.
• Add green onions and bell pepper into the eggs and stir to mix well.
• Add egg mixture over chorizo.
• Bake for 45 to 50 mins. until the top is golden brown.
• Place cilantro on top.

NUTRITIONAL INFORMATION:

Calories   750
Fat   58g
Carbohydrates   7g
Protein   48g
Sodium   2210mg

Paleo Beef Fajitas Skillet

INGREDIENTS:

Steak:
⅛ tsp. cumin
⅛ tsp. ground black pepper
⅛ tsp. paprika
¼ tsp. ground black pepper
¼ tsp. of ground cayenne red pepper
½ tsp. chili powder
½ tsp. dried oregano
½ tsp. Sea salt
1 lime juiced
1½ pound flank steak, sliced into thin ribbons

Vegetables:
¼ cup chopped cilantro
1 cup vegetable broth
1 de-seeded and sliced red bell pepper, trimmed
1 de-seeded and sliced yellow bell pepper, trimmed
1 minced garlic clove
1 peeled and sliced into thin slices yellow onion, trimmed
1 thinly sliced avocado, peeled and seeded
1 thinly sliced jalapeno, seeded
2 sliced green onions, green part
2 tbsp. organic coconut oil
5 oz. shitake mushrooms

DIRECTIONS:

•In a large bowl combine spices, steak and lime juice and toss together until steak is coated completely. Put aside.
•Over med-high heat, heat a large heavy skillet. Add coconut oil and add the steak.
•Lay the steak out so it will be in a single layer on pan.

•Sear the steak for 3 to 4 minutes, flip to cook the other side for 3 to 4 minutes more. Make sure that the outside is completely seared. Transfer the steak on the plate and set aside.

•Add peppers, mushrooms, onions and garlic to pan toss to coat. Make sure there is enough juice from the steak to coat your veggies. You can add ¼ cup of veggie broth if needed.

•Scrape any excess brown bits at the bottom of the pan. Toss your vegetables until it soften or for around 15 minutes.

•Add the jalapeno, steak, green onion, veggie broth and juices that you collected on the plate. Toss and cook for another 5 to 8 minutes.

•Turn off heat, garnish it with cilantro, slice of avocado and jalapeno slices if you want.

•Serve together with fajitas.

NUTRITIONAL INFORMATION:

Calories   322
Fat   19.4g
Carbohydrates   12.4g
Protein   26.5g
Sodium   277.3mg

Paleo Turkey Bacon Meatballs With Tomato Sauce

INGREDIENTS:

1 (8-ounce) pack finely chopped fresh mushrooms
1 large chopped onion
1 large egg, lightly beaten
1 tablespoon Italian seasoning
2 (14.5-ounce) cans fire-roasted diced tomatoes
2 pound lean ground turkey
2 tablespoon coconut oil
4 slices bacon

DIRECTIONS:
•On a paper towel-lined plate, place the bacon. Microwave the bacon for 1 ½ to 2 mins. on high. Crumble the bacon.
•In a medium size bowl, combine mushrooms, egg, ground turkey, onion, bacon and Italian seasoning. Shape the mixture into meatballs.
•Heat a nonstick skillet over medium heat. Add oil. Cook meatballs until brown and there is no pink in the center or for four minutes with frequent stirring.
•Remove from the pan, and keep warm.
•Add tomatoes into the pan let it boil and simmer for 15 mins. or until thickens.
•Add the cooked meatballs into the pan with tomatoes and simmer for around 5 minutes or until heated through.

NUTRITIONAL INFORMATION:
Calories   380
Fat   26g
Carbohydrates   3g
Protein   30g
Sodium   310mg

Yummy Paleo Spaghetti Squash With Pancetta

INGREDIENTS:

1 3 ounce pack pancetta, diced
1 diced bell pepper
2 small or 1 large shallots, finely diced
1 teaspoon Coconut Secret Garlic Sauce
1 large spaghetti squash, prepared

DIRECTIONS:
•In a big skillet cook the pancetta over medium heat.
•Add shallots and bell pepper as soon as the fat has rendered. Partially cover the pan and cook, stir occasionally until the veggies have softened and the shallot is translucent.
•Remove the cover and increase the heat slightly. To add a golden brown color to the veggies, continue cooking for a several minutes more.
•Add the spaghetti squash and garlic sauce. Stir and cook for several minutes to make it even more flavorful. Serve.

NUTRITIONAL INFORMATION:

Calories   260
Fat   15g
Carbohydrates   35g
Protein   8g
Sodium   270mg

Healthy Roasted Chicken With Lemon & Sage

INGREDIENTS:

2 tablespoon of ghee or unsalted butter
1 1/2 pounds skin on, bone in chicken breast

1 bunch coarsely chopped fresh sage
1 lemon sliced
Sea salt & pepper to taste

DIRECTIONS:

•Pre-heat your oven to 450 degrees Fahrenheit.
•Form a pocket between the meat and the skin.
•Melt the butter and spread it under the skin. Add sage, pepper, lemon slices, and salt.
•Rub with softened butter the outside part of the chicken and season with pepper and salt.
•Put the chicken on the rack and roast until the meat is cooked completely and the skin is golden brown for 30 to 35 minutes.

NUTRITIONAL INFORMATION:

Calories   250
Fat   10g
Carbohydrates   5g
Protein   36g
Sodium   390mg
Fiber   2g

Paleo Burger With Spinach And Sun-Dried Tomato

INGREDIENTS:

⅛ tsp. Black Pepper
⅛ tsp. Sea Salt
1 ½ c. chop Spinach
1 c. drain and chop Sun-Dried Tomatoes in Olive Oil
1 lb. Ground Beef
2 tbsp. Coconut Oil

DIRECTIONS:

•With your hands, combine all the ingredients in a big bowl. Shape the meat mixture into patties.
•In a frying pan, melt coconut oil over med-high heat. Adjust heat to medium and continue cooking the patties for 4 to 5 minutes on each side, or until cooked through. Serve.

NUTRITIONAL INFORMATION:

Calories   340
Fat   24g
Carbohydrates   9g
Protein   24g
Sodium   370mg
Fiber   2g

Crispy Paleo Homemade Chicken Nuggets

INGREDIENTS:

¼ cup ghee or coconut oil for frying
¼ teaspoon black pepper
1 and ½ - 2 c. blanched almond flour
1 egg, whisked
1 pound chicken tenderloins
1 teaspoon fine grain sea salt
1 teaspoon onion powder
1 teaspoon smoked paprika

DIRECTIONS:

•Cut the chicken into 1 to 2 inch bite size and put aside.
•Combine smoked paprika, black pepper, almond flour, onion powder, and salt in a shallow bowl and mix well.
•In another bowl, whisk the egg.
•Over medium fire, heat a large cast iron pan and add ghee or coconut oil. Make sure the oil is hot enough (drop a bit of almond flour and see if it sizzles) before adding the chicken.
•Dredge several chicken slices at a time. First coat the chicken in egg, then dredge it in almond flour mixture remove extra mixture. Then add it into hot pan.
•Cook the chicken until cooked through or for 2 to 4 minutes on each side.
•Most likely, you will need to fry in 2 batches. To prevent it from burning, adjust the heat and add more oil to the pan if needed for the next batch.
•Transfer into a dish lined with paper towel to remove excess oil. Serve hot.

NUTRITIONAL INFORMATION:

Calories   240
Fat   15g
Carbohydrates   1g
Protein   26g

Sodium	740mg
Fiber	0g

Paleo Coconut Butternut Squash Curry

INGREDIENTS:

1 can coconut milk (unsweetened)
1 red pepper
1 tablespoon coconut oil
1 tablespoon Garam masala
1 teaspoon cinnamon
1 teaspoon coriander
2 ½ cups shredded or cubed chicken
2 cups butternut squash
2 teaspoon dry onions
2 teaspoon turmeric
2 teaspoons melted coconut oil for roasting squash
Salt and Pepper to taste
Sprinkle of salt, cinnamon and pepper for roasting squash
Toppings: unsweetened shredded coconut, chopped cashew pieces and cilantro

DIRECTIONS:

•Pre-heat your oven to 450 degrees Fahrenheit.
•Peel the squash and cut into half. Remove the seeds and cut into small cubes. •Combine with salt, coconut oil, pepper and sprinkle some cinnamon.
•On a baking sheet lined with foil spread squash and roast it for 20 to 30 mins., or until tender but not too soft.
•Meanwhile, cook chicken and cut into cubes or shred it.
•Dice red peppers and saute it using coconut oil until soft.
•Add the spices and stir to coat peppers, cook until very fragrant or for about 1 to 2 minutes.
•Add coconut milk and simmer for 4 to 5 mins.
•Add butternut squash and chicken and keep it warm.
•Top with shredded coconut, chopped cashew pieces and cilantro.

NUTRITIONAL INFORMATION:

Calories   570
Fat   39g
Carbohydrates   31g
Protein   34g
Sodium   530mg
Fiber   9g

Paleo Puerto Rican Style Lasagna

INGREDIENTS:

1 pound breakfast sausage
2-4 tablespoon neutral-flavored oil
3 c. peeled and cubed jicama
4 large plantains, very ripe
6 large eggs
8 ounce chopped spinach (fresh or frozen)
Salt to taste

DIRECTIONS:
•Over medium heat, heat a large skillet and add 2 tablespoon of flavored oil.
•Prepare the plantain, peel and slice it lengthwise into ¼ inch thick slices.
•Fry in batches the plantain until caramelized and golden brown. You can add more oil half way of the cooking process if needed. Put aside.
•Pre-heat the oven to 350 degrees Fahrenheit.
•Use the same skillet in cooking the jicama and sausage until sausage becomes brown.
•Add the spinach and cook for 2 to 3 minutes or until wilted. Turn off the heat. •Add salt if needed.
•Oil an 8 x 8 baking pan and cover the lower part of the dish with one layer of plantains.
•On top of the plantains add ½ of the sausage mixture. Cover it with another layer of plantain. Repeat the procedure until you consume all the sausage mixture and plantains.
•Whisk together the eggs and add it into the lasagna. Bake for 30 to 35 minutes until the egg is cooked well. Let it stand for 10 minutes before cutting and serving.

NUTRITIONAL INFORMATION:
Calories   220
Fat   4.5g

Carbohydrates   39g
Protein   8g
Sodium   200mg

Healthy Paleo Salmon Cakes Recipe

INGREDIENTS:

1 egg
1 small sweet potato
1 tsp. pepper
1 tsp. salt
1/2 tsp. paprika
2 tbsp. fresh or dried parsley
2 tbsp. melted coconut oil, (for brushing)
2 thinly sliced scallions
3 (6 ounce) cans wild caught salmon (boneless)

DIRECTIONS:

•Pre-heat your oven to 425 degrees Fahrenheit. Drain the canned salmon.
•Microwave the sweet potato for 2 minutes or until tender and can be cut easily. •Don't forget to poke holes on it before placing it in the microwave.
•In a big bowl, combine the egg, parsley, pepper, salmon, scallions, dill and paprika.
•Slice the sweet potato in half and remove the skin. Allow it to cool down and then add it into the salmon mix.
•Use parchment paper to line a baking sheet, brush melted coconut oil on it.
•Scoop 1/3 cup of salmon mixture and place it on the baking sheet. Flatten into half inch thick, make sure that the thickness is even throughout.
•Bake for 20 mins. then flip and cook for another 10 mins. or until the patties start to brown or cooked through.
•Serve together with tartar sauce or with English muffins.

NUTRITIONAL INFORMATION:

Calories   260
Fat   12g
Carbohydrates   8g
Protein   28g
Sodium   720mg
Fiber   2g

Paleo Fried Chicken Dipped In Shredded Coconut

INGREDIENTS:
1 pound boneless and skinless chicken breasts
1 egg
2 tablespoon coconut oil
Sea salt to taste
Crushed red pepper to taste
1/2 teaspoon garlic powder
1/4 c. coconut flour
1/4 c. unsweetened shredded coconut

DIRECTIONS:
•Combine shredded coconut, red pepper, coconut flour, sea salt and garlic powder in a bowl.
•In another bowl beat the egg.
•Dip the chicken breast into the beaten egg, then roll it in the dry mixture until completely covered.
•Over medium heat, heat a frying pan and add the coconut oil.
•Fry the chicken until it is cooked through. For bigger chicken breast the coating will start to brown before it is fully cooked.
•Remove the chicken and place it in the baking sheet at 350 degrees Fahrenheit for 5 to 10 minutes. Cover the chicken with foil when baking or you can bake the chicken for 25 mins. at 400 degrees Fahrenheit. Make sure not to over bake the chicken.

NUTRITIONAL INFORMATION:
Calories   240
Fat   13g
Carbohydrates   4g
Protein   26g
Sodium   360mg
Fiber   1g

Paleo Coconut Lemon Chicken Curry

INGREDIENTS:

1 can full fat coconut milk
1 tablespoon curry spice
1 teaspoon turmeric
1/2 teaspoon sea salt
6 ethically raised chicken breasts or thighs
zest and juice from 1 lemon

DIRECTIONS:

•Set your crock pot or slow cooker into high heat
•Place all the ingredients into the slow cooker
•Cook for four hours
•Serve warm.

NUTRITIONAL INFORMATION:

Calories   440
Fat   29g
Carbohydrates   10g
Protein   40g
Sodium   380mg
   Fiber   4g

Tasty Paleo Deconstructed Cabbage Roll Soup

INGREDIENTS:

1 1/2 pound ground beef
1 cup diced onion
1 large head cabbage, halved and sliced
1 teaspoon black pepper
1/2 pound ground pork
1/2 teaspoon dried thyme
2 cans diced tomatoes, drained
2 tablespoon butter
2 tablespoon fresh parsley, chopped
2 tablespoon olive oil
2 teaspoon garlic powder
2 teaspoon onion powder
2 teaspoon sea salt
2 teaspoon smoked paprika
3 cups riced cauliflower
3 teaspoon dried oregano
4 cloves minced garlic
6 ounce can tomato paste
6 cups beef stock

DIRECTIONS:

•Place the olive oil and butter in a Dutch oven or huge stock pot over medium heat.
•Add the garlic and onion. Cook until the garlic is fragrant and onion is translucent.
•Add the ground pork and ground beef to the pan. Cook until golden brown and remove any excess oil.
•Add the oregano, garlic powder, beef broth, paprika, onion powder, sea salt, tomato paste, cabbage, black pepper, parsley, thyme, riced cauliflower and tomatoes.

•Boil and then lower the heat and simmer for 30 to 45 mins.

NUTRITIONAL INFORMATION:

Calories   265
Fat   15g
Carbohydrates   11.5g
Protein   19g
Fiber   4g

Paleo Baked Avocado Sticks Recipe

INGREDIENTS:

⅓ cup arrowroot (tapioca) flour
½ tsp. black pepper
½ tsp. fine sea salt
1 large egg, beaten
1 tbsp. water
1 tsp. onion powder
1 tsp. paprika
1 tsp. stone ground mustard
1-1/2 c. crushed pork rinds
2 ripe but firm avocados, pits removed
2 tsp. garlic powder

DIRECTIONS:

•Pre-heat your oven to 425 degrees Fahrenheit, and use foil to line a baking sheet.
•Cut the avocado in half and remove the pit.
•Slice each half into 3 or 4 slices, and put aside.
•Prepare 3 bowls for the dipping stations. First bowl - combine the arrowroot and ½ of the seasonings. Second bowl- combine water, beaten egg and mustard. •Third bowl- mix the pork rinds with the remaining seasonings.
•Dip the slices of avocado in the following order – arrowroot dip then egg dip and then the pork dip. Place them on the baking sheet.
•Bake the avocado fries for around 10 to 12 minutes, then flip and then continue baking for another 2 to 4 minutes.
•Serve warm and fresh from the oven.
 NUTRITIONAL INFORMATION:

Calories   260
Fat   22g

Carbohydrates   17g
Protein   6g
Sodium   250mg
Fiber   10g

Paleo Cinco De Mayo Burgers Recipe

INGREDIENTS:

⅓ c. fresh cilantro, finely chopped
½ c. red bell pepper, finely chopped
½ teaspoon black pepper
½finely chopped jalapeno pepper, seeds and white inner membrane removed
¾ c. onion, finely chopped
1 teaspoon onion powder
1 teaspoon sea salt
1-1/2 pound grass fed ground beef
2 cloves garlic, finely chopped
2 tablespoon ghee or avocado oil

DIRECTIONS:

•Place all the ingredients in a big bowl. Use your hands to mix all the ingredients until well combined.
•Portion the meat using a 1/3 cup measuring cup. Fill the cup with the meat mixture and then turn the meat out and form it into patties. To keep the patties flat, press your thumb in the center.
•Over med-high heat, heat a large skillet and add 2 tbsp. of avocado oil or ghee until it shimmers. Fry the patties for four minutes on one side, flip and then fry for another two to three minutes depending on how thick your patties and your preferred doneness.
•Serve together with lettuce leaves or green cabbage and top with fresh cilantro, salsa, guacamole, fresh tomato and others.

NUTRITIONAL INFORMATION:

Calories   290
Fat   20g
Carbohydrates   3g
Protein   22g
Sodium   280mg

Fiber   1g

Paleo Fresh Spring Rolls With Umami Mayo Dip Recipe

INGREDIENTS:

1 large bunch of collard greens
1 thinly sliced carrot
½ cucumber, seeds removed and thinly sliced
2 thinly sliced green onions, dark green tops removed
1 bunch of fresh mint, cilantro or basil leaves
1 pack kelp noodles, optional
¼ cup of Umami Mayo for dipping
6-7 medium-sized raw shrimp

DIRECTIONS:

•Blanch the collard leaves to loss its bitter flavor and make it pliable.
Prepare a large bowl with ice water. Boil water in a very large pot.
•Dip the entire collard leaves into the boiling water for one minute. Then place them right away in the ice water to cool and stop the cooking process. Remove the water and put aside.
•Devein the shrimp if you want. In a small skillet over medium heat, add two to three tablespoons of water and the raw shrimp. Cover and cook until the shrimps are pink or for around 2 mins. Allow it to cool down. Slice the shrimp in half from heat to tail.
•Wash and drain the kelp noodles. Put aside.
•Prepare the green onion, cucumber and carrot. Slice them thinly.
•Remove the tough stem of the collard leaves using a sharp knife by cutting it upward toward the top of the leaf. To make the leaves roll better make an upside down V shape.

•To assemble the wrap: place the collard leaf on a flat surface. At top of the leaf place two halves of shrimp. Then place a small amount of the noodles on top of the shrimp..
•Roll and wrap like burrito. Slowly but apply pressure, and roll the shrimp toward the end of the stem.
•Once you have completed the first roll continue with the remaining ingredients.
•Divide each wrap into 2 and serve cold with your favorite dip.

NUTRITIONAL INFORMATION:

Calories   110
Fat   5g
Carbohydrates   13g
Protein   5g
Sodium   150mg
Fiber   4g

Paleo Banana Beef Pie

INGREDIENTS:

¼ c. tomato sauce
⅓ c. diced red pepper
½ diced onion
½ tsp. achiote or paprika
½ tsp. black pepper
½ tsp. sea salt
1 bay leaf
1 c. fire-roasted diced tomatoes
1 lb. grass-fed ground beef
1 tbsp. apple cider vinegar
1 tbsp. water
2 tbsp. chopped olives (green or black)
2 tbsp. dried currants (or raisins)
3 eggs
4 oz. can diced mild green chilis
4–5 large, slightly ripe bananas (some yellow, some dark spots)
Chopped cilantro for garnish, optional
Coconut oil for frying

DIRECTIONS:

•Pre- heat your oven to 350 degrees Fahrenheit. Put some oil in an 8 x 8 baking pan with oil and put aside.
•Over med-high heat, heat a large skillet. Cook the ground beef completely until golden brown.
•Reduce the heat and using the same skillet, add the onion, bay leaf and red pepper.
•Preheat the oven to 350°F (175°C). Grease the inside of an 8" x 8" baking dish with coconut oil and set aside.
•Continue cooking for 4 to 5 minutes until the vegetables are softened.

•Add the diced tomatoes, olives, green chilis, tomato sauce, paprika, pepper, currants, salt, apple cider vinegar and olives. Stir to mix well and simmer for ten more minutes.

•Meanwhile, peel and slice the plantains into 1/3 diagonal pieces. In peeling, remove both ends and cut through the skin lengthwise, then peel off in sections. •In case there are still some skin remains, cut it off using a knife.

•In another pan over medium heat, add coconut oil and start to brown the bananas in a single layer for around 2 mins. on each side.

•You need to do this a few time until all the bananas are golden brown.

•Once cooked, transfer into a plate lined with paper towel to drain.

•Whisk the eggs and water in a small bowl.

•Assemble the pie. Spread half of the meat and veggie mixture in the bottom of the dish.

•Pour 1/3 of the beaten egg. Place the bananas in a single layer on top of the egg. •Do the same layering and top with the rest of the beaten egg.

•Bake for 45 mins. or until the eggs are set. Allow it to stand for another 10 mins. before slicing it.

NUTRITIONAL INFORMATION:

Calories   560
Fat   22g
Carbohydrates   65g
Protein   30g
Sodium   540mg
Fiber   6g

Spicy Paleo Jalapeño Crab Dip For Veggie Sticks

INGREDIENTS:

¼ c. Brazil nuts
⅓ c. almond meal
½ c. chopped pickled jalapeño rings
½ c. homemade mayo
1 clove garlic
1 tablespoon coconut oil or ghee
1 teaspoon gluten-free Worcestershire sauce
1 teaspoon hot sauce
16 ounce high-quality canned crabmeat
2 cloves finely chopped garlic

DIRECTIONS:

•Pre-heat your oven to 350 degrees Fahrenheit.
•Place one garlic clove and Brazil nuts in a food processor and pulse until fluffy and in fine bits form.
•In a small casserole dish or oven proof glass bowl, combine the chopped garlic, mayo, crab, chopped jalapeno, hot sauce, Brazil nuts mixture, and Worcestershire sauce. Stir until well mixed. Add the sea salt to taste.
•Over medium heat, heat a small skillet. Add 1 tablespoon coconut oil or ghee and almond meal. Stir until the almond meal becomes toasty and golden brown. •Make sure not to leave it for it can burn easily.
•Place the almond meal crumbs on top of the crap mixture. Bake for 30 mins. or until hot and bubbly.

NUTRITIONAL INFORMATION:

Calories   230
Fat   16g
Carbohydrates   8g

Protein   16g
Sodium   380mg
Fiber   2g

Nutritious Acorn Squash Stuffed With Ground Beef Recipe

INGREDIENTS:

¼ teaspoon nutmeg
½ teaspoon cinnamon
½ teaspoon sea salt
1 apple, any variety
1 large acorn squash
1 lb. ground beef
1 onion
1 tablespoon chopped fresh rosemary
1 teaspoon black pepper
1 teaspoon ground sage
2 teaspoon dried thyme
2 teaspoon fennel seeds
6 slices bacon

DIRECTIONS:

•Pre-heat your oven to 375 degrees Fahrenheit. Use parchment paper or foil to line the baking dish.
•Cut the squash in half and remove the seeds out. Place it on the baking sheet and roast until the flesh is soft, around 45 mins. Remove and allow it to cool down to touch.
•Meanwhile, prepare the stuffing. Dice the apple and cut the onion into medium size pieces.
•Slice the bacon into small pieces.
•In a big skillet brown the bacon over medium heat. Add the onion and cook for 5 to 10 mins. or until translucent and soft.
•Add the apples and cook for another 5 to 10 mins.
•Transfer the bacon, apple and onion mixture to a big bowl.
•Heat again the same skillet over med-high heat, and cook the ground beef until it becomes golden brown. Remove the excess oil in case it yielded a lot of oil.

•Add the herbs and spices – fennel seeds, nutmeg, rosemary, salt, thyme, sage, cinnamon and pepper.
•Add the ground beef into the same big bowl. Stir to mix well.
•Use a spoon to scoop out some of the flesh of the squash and add it into the beef.
•Fill the squash boats with the beef mixture.
•Place the squash boats in the oven and bake for another 15 mins. at 375 degrees Fahrenheit until heated through.

NUTRITIONAL INFORMATION:

Calories	600
Fat	41g
Carbohydrates	25g
Protein	32g
Sodium	830mg
Fiber	5g

Chapter 6: 20 Paleo Snack Recipes

The most important thing about paleo diet is that you are not forbidden to eat the foods that you want. You just need to cut them out or replace some ingredients with healthful alternatives. It means that you need to stay away from pre-packaged snack foods that you will find in the supermarket. Preparing your own snack is the best way to ensure yourself that you are eating natural foods. Here are some interesting and delicious recipes that you can prepare.

Paleo Crispy Banana Chips

INGREDIENTS:

2 green plantains
3 tablespoon coconut oil
Sea salt to taste

DIRECTIONS:

•Place coconut oil in a large frying pan and heat over medium heat.
•Peel your plantains and cut them into thin slices around 3 to 4 mm.
•Place the banana slices into the pan, make sure that they will not overlap with each other.
•Cook for about 4 to 5 minutes on one side or until golden brown and then flip and cook for another few minutes until golden brown.
•Sprinkle sea salt before removing from the heat.
•Remove from the pan and allow it to cool down for a few minutes.
•Serve.

NUTRITIONAL INFORMATION:

Calories   200
Fat   10g
Carbohydrates   29g
Fiber   2g
Protein   1g
Sodium   200mg

Healthy Paleo Cherry And Cashew Snack Bars

INGREDIENTS:

¼ c. quality dark chocolate
¼ c. roughly chopped pumpkin seeds
¼ tsp. sea salt
⅓ c. almond flour
⅓ c. honey
½ c. finely chopped dried cherries
1 tbsp. almond butter
1 tsp. vanilla
1⅓ c. roughly chopped cashews

DIRECTIONS:

•Pre-heat your oven to 300 degrees Fahrenheit. Use parchment paper to line an 8 inch baking pan, let the ends drape on the pan sides.
•Combine almond butter, vanilla, honey, sea salt, and almond flour in a medium bowl. Use spatula to blend it well.
•Fold in the pumpkin seeds, cashews and cherries and mix until distributed evenly.
•Press the mixture into the prepared baking pan, spread it in the corners. The bars should be around ½ inch thick.
•Bake for 22 to 24 minutes at 300 degrees Fahrenheit.
•Cool the pan. Place it in the fridge to cool it down further before slicing it into bars. Drizzle some melted chocolate on top.
•Wrap it individually in the fridge or freezer.

NUTRITIONAL INFORMATION:

Calories   460
Fat   31g
Carbohydrates   39g

Fiber	3g
Protein	13g
Sodium	110mg

Complete Paleo Snack Balls

INGREDIENTS:

1 c. Macadamia Nuts
1/2 c. dried Pineapple
1/2 c. dried Mango
1/2 c. Shredded Coconut
1/2 c. Shredded Coconut for dipping
1/8 teaspoon Sea Salt

DIRECTIONS:

•Combine the fruits in a food processor and process until it is thick enough to make a ball.
•Add the nuts, sea salt and shredded coconut to the food processor and process until well blended.
•Get a walnut-sized amount and using your hands roll it to make a ball. Dip into the reserve shredded coconut and coat evenly.

NUTRITIONAL INFORMATION:

Calories   170
Fat   4g
Carbohydrates   13g
Fiber   2g
Protein   1g
Sodium   55mg

Easy-To-Do Crispy Kale Chips For Snack

INGREDIENTS:

2 tablespoon olive oil
1 bunch washed and dried kale
Salt to taste

DIRECTIONS:

•Pre-heat your oven to 300 degrees Fahrenheit. Discard the center stems and either cut or tear up the leaves.
•Toss the olive oil and kale together in a big bowl, sprinkle it with salt. Place them in the baking sheet.
•Bake them for 15 mins. or until crispy at 300 degrees Fahrenheit.

NUTRITIONAL INFORMATION:

Calories   230
Fat   16g
Carbohydrates   23g
Fiber   5g
Protein   7g
Sodium   490mg

Crispy Butternut Squash Spiced Chips

INGREDIENTS:

1 medium butternut squash
2 tablespoon extra virgin coconut oil, melted
3 to 6 drops liquid Stevia extract (optional)
Salt to taste
1 teaspoon gingerbread spice mix (ingredients- ½ tsp cinnamon, small amount of nutmeg, cloves, allspice and ginger)

DIRECTIONS:

•Prepare the gingerbread spice mix – combine ½ teaspoon cinnamon, ginger, pinch of nutmeg, cloves and allspice.
•Pre-heat your oven to 250 degrees Fahrenheit. Remove the butternut squash peel and use mandolin to slice thinly. If you don't have mandolin make sure that the slices are not more than 1/8 inch thin. Place the butternut in a bowl.
•Combine melted coconut oil, stevia, and gingerbread spice mix in a small bowl.
•Add the oil mixture in the butternut squash and combine well to coat evenly.
•Arrange the butternut slices close to each other on the baking tray with parchment paper.
•Place it in the oven and cook for 1 ½ hour or until crispy. You can spray coconut oil half way through to make it crispier.
•Once done, take it out of the oven and store in an air-tight container.

NUTRITIONAL INFORMATION:

Calories   373
Fat   6.9g
Carbohydrates   12.4g
Fiber   2.5g
Protein   1g

Sodium   0mg

Crispy Baked Apple With Cinnamon Chips

INGREDIENTS:

1 teaspoon cinnamon
1-2 apples

DIRECTIONS:

•Pre-heat your oven to 200 degrees Fahrenheit.
•Use a mandolin or sharp knife to slice the apples thinly. Remove the seeds.
•Use parchment paper in the baking sheet and arrange the apple slices make sure that it will not overlap each other.
•Sprinkle cinnamon on top of the apple.
•Bake for one hour, then flip. Bake for another hour, flip occasionally until all the apple slices are dry.
•Store in a tightly closed container.

NUTRITIONAL INFORMATION:

Calories   35
Fat   0g
Carbohydrates   10g
Fiber   1g
Protein   0g
Sodium   0mg

Paleo Zucchini Rolls With Tomatoes And Bacon

INGREDIENTS:

½ cup fresh basil
½ cup sun-dried tomatoes, drained
1 cup soft goat cheese
14 thin slices streaky bacon
3 small or baby zucchini, organic
    4 tablespoon raspberry vinegar or any other fruit vinegar

DIRECTIONS:

•Pre-heat your oven to 400 degree Fahrenheit. Slice into thin strips the zucchini using a peeler.
•Place in a mixing bowl and add 4 tbsp. of raspberry vinegar. Make sure that the zucchini are covered with vinegar. Allow it to stand for 10 mins.
•Slice the bacon lengthwise and place on a lined baking tray or rack.
•Bake for 5 mins. or until slightly crispy.
•Take it out of the oven and put a bacon strip on each zucchini slice. Put goat cheese on top, freshly chopped basil and a small piece of sun-dried tomato.
•Wrap the zucchini rolls and place a toothpick on each one of them.
•Enjoy.

NUTRITIONAL INFORMATION:
Calories   78
Fat   19.2g
Carbohydrates   6.3g
Fiber   1.3g
Protein   15.7g
Sodium   0mg

Paleo Bacon And Artichoke With Spinach And Blue Cheese Dip

INGREDIENTS:

1 1/2 tablespoon olive oil
1 can artichoke hearts, remove the liquid (reserve 1/2 tablespoon)
1/2 c. cashews
1/2 tablespoon artichoke juice
1/4 teaspoon dry mustard
2 large handfuls baby spinach
1/2 teaspoon garlic powder
3 ounce blue cheese
1/2 teaspoon onion powder
Salt and pepper to taste
3 slices bacon

DIRECTIONS:

•Place the bacon in a skillet and cook over medium heat. Once done place on a paper towels and set aside.
•Cut the artichoke hearts in half lengthwise. In the same skillet where you cook the bacon saute spinach and warm the artichoke hearts. Allow it to cool down.
•Place cashews in a blender and pulse until a fine powder is produced.
•Drizzle olive oil and the reserved artichoke juice.
•Add half of the artichoke spinach mixture and season. Pulse again a couple times to mix well but not liquefy.
•In a bowl, combine blended ingredients, the remaining artichoke and spinach, crumbled blue cheese and chopped bacon.
•Serve together with sweet potato chips.
•Enjoy.

NUTRITIONAL INFORMATION:

Calories   420
Fat   33g
Carbohydrates   19g
Fiber   7g
Protein   15g
Sodium   710mg

Pumpkin And Banana With Almond Butter Snack Bars

INGREDIENTS:

1 (150 grams) ripe banana
1 cup (250 grams) pumpkin puree or cooled roast pumpkin
1 tsp. cinnamon
1 tsp. vanilla
1/2 cup almond butter
3 cups finely shredded desiccated coconut
Pinch of salt

DIRECTIONS:

•Pre-heat the oven to 350^0F.
•Grease a lined 20 x 20 square cake tin using baking paper, hang over the sides for easy removal.
•In your food processor or blender add all the ingredients and blend to mix well.
•Place the mixture into the tin and bake for 30 mins. or until golden on top and when the skewer comes out clean when inserted.
•Take it out of the oven and let it stand for 5 mins. and then slowly move the slice into a cooling rack.
•Cut it into bars when cooled down.
•Enjoy.

NUTRITIONAL INFORMATION:

Calories   260
Fat   18g
Carbohydrates   21g
Fiber   5g
Protein   6g
Sodium   230mg

Sweet Paleo Honey Pumpkin Seed Clusters

INGREDIENTS:

1 teaspoon vanilla extract
2 teaspoon coconut sugar
2 teaspoon honey
Boiled water
1/2 cup pumpkin seeds

DIRECTIONS:

•Pre-heat your oven to 300 degrees Fahrenheit.
•Combine coconut sugar, vanilla and honey in a medium bowl. Stir to produce a thick paste and add a small drop of water at a time to thin it out and produce runny syrup.
•Add the pumpkin seeds and stir well to coat them evenly.
•Scoop a generous amount of the pumpkin seeds in the baking sheet, repeat the procedure until you used up all the mixture and cook for 15 to 20 mins. until the clusters become brown.
•Remove it from the oven and allow it to stand for a few minutes to cool down. As soon as the mixture cooled a little bit you press the clusters together so they won't fall apart. They will dry easily.
•You can eat it on their own or you can add it on top of your cereal.

NUTRITIONAL INFORMATION:

Calories   25
Fat   2g
Carbohydrates   1g
Fiber   0g
Protein   1g
Sodium   0mg

Paleo Maple Roasted Parsnip Chips

INGREDIENTS:

500g Parsnips
3 tbsp. Maple Syrup
1/4 c. melted Coconut Oil

DIRECTIONS:

•Pre-heat your oven to 392 degrees Fahrenheit.
•Peel the parsnips and cut them into thin slices and place them in an oven proof dish.
•Add coconut oil on top of the parsnip and coat evenly.
•Drizzle maple syrup on top and stir to mix well.
•Bake for 15 mins. take it out of the oven and flip the parsnips to bake the other side.
•Return it in the oven and cook for another 10 to 15 mins. or until golden brown.
•Once done take it out of the oven and allow it to cool down before serving.

NUTRITIONAL INFORMATION:

Calories   147.1
Fat   2.1g
Carbohydrates   32.3g
Fiber   3.7g
Protein   2.1g
Sodium   53mg

Paleo Hemp And Pistachios Bars

INGREDIENTS:

½ teaspoon spirulina powder
1/2 c. pistachios
1/2 c. pumpkin seeds
1/4 c. orange juice
1/4 c. hemp hearts
1/4 c. coconut oil
3/4 c. shredded coconut
3/4 c. chopped dates

DIRECTIONS:

•Combine all the ingredients in a food processor and pulse until the mixture is crumbly and stick together.
•Transfer into an 8 inch glass dish or cake pan and press.
•Place in the fridge for an hour and slice.
•Serve.

NUTRITIONAL INFORMATION:

Calories   320
Fat   22g
Carbohydrates   29g
Fiber   4g
Protein   6g
Sodium   30mg

Paleo Rosemary And Sweet Potato Chips

INGREDIENTS:

1 tablespoon melted coconut oil
1 teaspoon sea salt
2 large sweet potatoes, peeled
2 teaspoon dried rosemary

DIRECTIONS:

•Pre-heat your oven to 375 degree Fahrenheit.
•Use mandolin to slice the sweet potatoes thinly.
•Grind rosemary and sea salt using mortar and pestle.
•Place sweet potatoes in a bowl and add the salt-seasoning mixture and coconut oil.
•Pour into a nonstick baking sheet and place it in the oven. After ten minutes take the dish out and flip the chips.
•Return it back in the oven and bake for another ten minutes.
•Take the pan out of the oven and place the chips that are starting to brown in the cooling rack.
•Return it back in the oven and bake for another 3 to 5 mins.
•Once done, place all the chips in the cooling rack.

NUTRITIONAL INFORMATION:

Calories   90
Fat   3.5g
Carbohydrates   13g
Fiber   2g
Protein   1g
Sodium   630mg

Paleo Coconut Date Balls Recipe

INGREDIENTS:

¼ c. ghee
½ c. raw honey
½ teaspoon sea salt
1 c. coconut flakes
1 cup roughly chopped dates
1 teaspoon vanilla extract
2 beaten eggs
2 c. chopped mixed nuts

DIRECTIONS:

•In a medium saucepan combine ghee, dates, eggs, and raw honey and place them over medium heat.
•Bring it to boil and stir occasionally, for 3 to 5 mins.
•Take it out of the heat and add in the vanilla stir and add the sea salt.
•Add the chopped nuts and stir until well mixed.
•Form the mixture into small balls.
•Roll the ball in the coconut flakes until completely coated.
•Place in the fridge until firm.

NUTRITIONAL INFORMATION:

Calories   110
Fat   5.7g
Carbohydrates   17.4g
Fiber   2.1g
Protein   2.3g
Sodium   1mg

Tasty Paleo White Bread Recipe

INGREDIENTS:

1 c. blanched almond meal
1 teaspoon baking soda
1/2 teaspoon coconut vinegar
1/2 teaspoon sea salt
1/4 c. ground flax
1/4 cup melted coconut oil
1/4 teaspoon stevia powder extract or 2 tablespoon honey
3 tablespoon sifted coconut flour
6 pastured eggs

DIRECTIONS:

•Pre-heat your oven to 350 degrees Fahrenheit.
•Use a parchment to line only the bottom of an 8 x 4 loaf pan.
•Beat the eggs, coconut oil, vinegar and sweetener in a large bowl until well mixed.
•In another bowl, mix the flax meal, almond meal, coconut flour, sea salt and baking soda stir until well mixed.
•Slowly add the dry ingredients into the wet ingredients make sure not to over stir it.
•Transfer the mixture in the lined loaf pan and bake for 35 to 40 mins.
•Take it out of the oven and allow it to cool down for around 12 mins.
•Pull up the parchment to remove the bread from the pan.
•Place the bread on a wire rack to cool down completely.
•Slice and enjoy.
•For leftovers you can store it in the fridge for a week.

NUTRITIONAL INFORMATION:

Calories   80
Fat   18.2g
Carbohydrates   6.2g

Fiber   3.6g
Protein   9.8g
Sodium   0mg

Paleo Sweet Potato Beef Burger With Avocado And Bacon Recipe

INGREDIENTS:

¼ teaspoon black pepper

¼ teaspoon salt

½ teaspoon baking soda

1 clove minced garlic

1 cup tapioca flour, divided, ⅓ and ⅔

1 egg

1 tablespoon fresh chopped dill

2 tablespoon avocado or olive oil divided

5 tablespoon water

DIRECTIONS:

•Pre-heat your oven to 350 degrees Fahrenheit.

•In a sauce pan combine 1 tablespoon olive oil with water and 1/3 cup of tapioca flour. Add in garlic and dill. Stir over low heat until it is thick enough to form a ball. Put aside and allow it to cool down.

•Combine the rest of the olive oil, baking soda, flour, salt and pepper in another bowl.

•Add the ball to the flour mixture and mix thoroughly.

•Knead the flour in until it turns into runny dough. It is important that you mix in the ball or you will get some jelly spots in your pita. If you want you can add some tapioca flour.

•Transfer the mixture into a baking sheet lined with parchment paper.

•Press the pitas with your wet hands as thin as possible. It is important that your hands are wet when working with the dough so it will not stick.

•Bake at 350 degrees Fahrenheit for 18 minutes, then flip over and bake for another 4 minutes on the other side.

NUTRITIONAL INFORMATION:

Calories   80
Fat   8g
Carbohydrates   0g
Fiber   0g
Protein   2g
Sodium   320mg

Paleo Crispy Pork Rinds Recipe

INGREDIENTS:

Pork skin
Salt

DIRECTIONS:

•Pre-heat the oven to 325 degrees Fahrenheit.
•Line a baking sheet with parchment paper and put the pork skin on it. Sprinkle some salt.
•Place the pork skin in the oven and bake for about 1 ½ hours to 3 hours or until crispy.
•Take it out of the oven and allow it to cool down a little bit. Serve.

NUTRITIONAL INFORMATION:

Calories   80
Fat   5g
Carbohydrates   0.0g
Fiber   0.0g
Protein   8g
    Sodium   330mg

Paleo Sweet Choco Coconut Macaroons

INGREDIENTS:

¼ c. of 100% pure cocoa powder
1 tsp. vanilla extract
2 tbsp. raw honey
3 c shredded coconut unsweetened
4 large egg whites
Dash of salt
Small dash of pure stevia

DIRECTIONS:

- Pre-heat your oven to 350 degrees Fahrenheit.
- Beat the egg whites using an electric whisker until peaks form.
- Add the stevia, vanilla extract, salt, honey and cocoa powder and mix well.
- Add in the shredded coconut.
- Bake for fifteen minutes.

NUTRITIONAL INFORMATION:

Calories	50
Fat	3g
Carbohydrates	7g
Fiber	1g
Protein	1g
Sodium	50mg

Healthy Almond Stuffed Dates Bacon Wrap

INGREDIENTS:

16 medium almonds, whole
16 medium dates
8 slices of bacon cut in half
Toothpick (optional)

DIRECTIONS:

•Pre-heat your oven to 375 degrees Fahrenheit.
•Use knife to open up the dates.
•Place almond on each date, and wrap half a bacon slice around it. Use toothpick to secure it if needed.
•Arrange the wrapped dates in a shallow baking sheet and bake with bacon seam down for around 7 mins.
•Flip and then bake for another 7 mins. or until the bacon becomes crispy.
•Serve cold or warm, and keep the leftovers in the fridge.

NUTRITIONAL INFORMATION:

Calories   44
Fat   1.5g
Carbohydrates   6.2g
Fiber   0.6g
Protein   1.5g
Sodium   87mg

Crispy Paleo Sugar-Free Coconut Flakes

INGREDIENTS:

¼ teaspoon Allspice
¼ teaspoon Nutmeg
¼ teaspoon Salt
1 c. Unsweetened Coconut Flakes
1 teaspoon Cinnamon
1 teaspoon melted Coconut Oil

DIRECTIONS:

•Pre-heat your oven to 350 degrees Fahrenheit. Use parchment paper to line a baking sheet.
•Place the coconut flakes in a Ziplock and add the nutmeg, salt, cinnamon and allspice. Shake to coat the flakes evenly.
•Add coconut oil in the bag and then shake again make sure all the flakes are coated evenly.
•Place the coconut flakes on the baking sheet and place in the oven on the center rack.
•Bake for three to five minute, keeping an eye all time to make sure it don't over burn.
•Take it out of the oven right away to prevent it from browning even further.

NUTRITIONAL INFORMATION:

Calories   110
Fat   10g
Carbohydrates   4g
Fiber   2g
Protein   1g
Sodium   0mg

Chapter 7: 19 Paleo Dessert And Smoothies Recipes

Your paleo lunch and dessert meal is not complete if you don't have dessert. There are some foods that are not part of the paleo plate, so make sure that you know what to serve for dessert. Don't stress yourself out, here some of the best paleo desserts and smoothies that you can serve to complete your paleo diet.

Nutritious Dates With Cashew Rolled In Shredded Coconut

INGREDIENTS:

¼ cup finely chopped raw cashews
14 large soft pitted Medjool dates
2 tbsp. coconut oil (at room temperature)
2 tbsp. raw cashew butter
A good pinch of sea salt
The seeds from half a vanilla bean
Unsweetened shredded organic coconut for rolling

DESCRIPTIONS:

•In a bowl of a food processor add coconut oil, salt, dates, vanilla bean seeds and cashew butter and process until smooth and can be form into a ball.
•Add in chopped cashews and refrigerate to make it firm for 10 mins.
•Slightly grease your hands and roll the date mixture to form a long rope and cut into small pieces.
•Put shredded coconut in a dish and roll the date in the coconut.
•Serve right away and refrigerate to make it firm and serve chilled.
•Store date rolls in an airtight container in the ref for 2 weeks.

NUTRITIONAL INFORMATION:

Calories   90
Fat   6g
Carbohydrates   8g
Fiber   1g
Protein   1g
Sodium   40mg

Yummy Paleo Chocolate Cupcakes

INGREDIENTS:

¼ c. cacao powder
¼ c. coconut flour
¼ c. coconut oil
¼ tsp. baking soda
¼ tsp. celtic sea salt
⅓ c. honey
4 large eggs

DIRECTIONS:

•Place all the dry and wet ingredients in a food processor and process until well mix.
•Use paper liners to line a muffin pan and scoop ¼ cup into each hole.
•Bake at 350 degrees Fahrenheit for 15 to 18 minutes.
•Cool and enjoy.

NUTRITIONAL INFORMATION:

Calories   140
Fat   9g
Carbohydrates   12g
Fiber   0g
Protein   3g
Sodium   115mg

Healthy Paleo Zucchini Brownies Without Flour

INGREDIENTS:

1 cup of almond butter
1 egg
1 teaspoon of vanilla
1 teaspoon of baking soda
1 teaspoon of cinnamon
1 cup of dark chocolate chips
1 1/2 cup zucchini shred them in a food processor.
1/2 teaspoon of nutmeg
1/3 cup of honey

DIRECTIONS:

•Pre-heat your oven to 350 degrees Fahrenheit.
•In a large bowl combine all the ingredients and mix well.
•Transfer into a greased 9 by 9 baking dish.
•Bake until the toothpick comes out clean or for 35 to 45 mins.

NUTRITIONAL INFORMATION:

Calories   570
Fat   42g
Carbohydrates   46g
Fiber   4g
Protein   12g
    Sodium   350mg

Sweet And Minty Paleo Peppermint Thin

INGREDIENTS:

⅛ tsp. celtic sea salt
¼ c. honey
¼ tsp. baking soda
½ tsp. peppermint extract
1 c. blanched almond flour
1 tsp. coconut flour
1 tsp. peppermint extract
2 tbsp. cacao powder
2 tbsp. palm shortening
6 oz. chocolate chunks

DIRECTIONS:

•Combine coconut flour, baking soda, almond flour, salt and cacao in a food processor.
•Pulse and add in honey, peppermint extract and shortening until dough forms.
•Line a baking pan using a parchment paper and roll out the dough to 1/8 inch thick.
•Freeze the dough for 15 mins.
•Cut the dough using a 2 inch cookie cutter.
•Place the cut cookies in the lined baking sheet.
•Bake at 350 degrees Fahrenheit for four minutes.
•Allow it to cool down completely on a baking pan and then freeze for one hour.
•Melt peppermint extract and chocolate in a small saucepan over low heat.
•Dip each cookie in chocolate, then arrange them on a parchment line plate.
•Refrigerate for one hour and serve.

NUTRITIONAL INFORMATION:

Calories   70
Fat   4g
Carbohydrates   9g
Fiber   1g
Protein   3g
Sodium   25mg

Pear And Parsley Smoothie Recipe

INGREDIENTS:

1 Thai coconut, meat and water
1/2 bunch parsley, stems cut
2 small cored pears,
3/4 cup peeled mango

DIRECTIONS:

•In your blender, add coconut meat and water first.
•Then add the mango and pears.
•Add the parsley last and blend on high until the smoothie is creamy or for 30 secs.

NUTRITIONAL INFORMATION:

Calories   454
Fat   4.3g
Carbohydrates   108.2g
Fiber   0g
Protein   5.7g
Sodium   0mg

Avocado And Spinach Paleo Smoothie With Strawberries

INGREDIENTS:

1 frozen ripe banana
1 cup fresh baby spinach, washed and dried
1 cup almond milk
1 tbsp. raw honey
1 tbsp. ground chia seeds
1/2 an avocado
    4-5 fresh strawberries

DIRECTIONS:

•In your blender add all the ingredients and blend for 30 seconds.
•Transfer into a tall glass or on a mason jar and serve.

NUTRITIONAL INFORMATION:

Calories   470
Fat   20g
Carbohydrates   67g
Fiber   12g
Protein   12g
Sodium   160mg

Paleo Avocado-Coconut Green Smoothie

INGREDIENTS:

1 large handful spinach
Sprinkle of vanilla extract
1/2 avocado
1/2 frozen banana
1-2 tablespoon coconut cream
1/4 c liquid egg whites (optional)
3/4 c coconut water

DIRECTIONS:

•Blend all the ingredients using your high speed blender with the liquids at the bottom and spinach on top.
•Blend for 30 seconds or until mixed thoroughly.
•Pour into serving glass and enjoy.

NUTRITIONAL INFORMATION:

Calories   360
Fat   26g
Carbohydrates   33g
Fiber   12g
Protein   6g
Sodium   210mg

Refreshing Paleo Fudge Pops Recipe

INGREDIENTS:

3/4 c. full fat coconut milk
1 avocado
2 tbsp. honey
1/4 c. cocoa powder, unsweetened
1 large banana
Pinch of salt
1 tsp. pure vanilla extract

DIRECTIONS:

•Pour all the ingredients in a food processor and process until smooth.
•Pour evenly into the popsicle molds.
•Place in the freezer for around 4 hours.
•Serve.

NUTRITIONAL INFORMATION:

Calories   90
Fat   6g
Carbohydrates   9g
Fiber   2g
Protein   1g
Sodium   30mg

Paleo Chocolate Chips Dessert

INGREDIENTS:

1 1/2 c. sifted blanched almond flour
1 whole egg
1/2 c. chocolate chips
1/2 tsp. vanilla extract
1/4 c. maple syrup
1/4 tsp. baking soda
1/4 tsp. sea salt
2 tbsp. melted coconut oil

DIRECTIONS:

•Let the maple syrup and egg stand at room temp. for about 30 mins.
•Combine all the dry ingredients in a bowl.
•Place the wet ingredients in another bowl and mix well.
•Add the wet ingredients mixture into the dry mixture and mix thoroughly.
•Add in the chocolate chips. Refrigerate for 30 minutes.
•Pre-heat the oven to 350 degrees Fahrenheit.
•On a cookie sheet lined with parchment paper spoon batter.
•Bake for 7 minutes. Press the top of the cookies using the back of the spatula. •Continue baking for another 5 minutes.
•Let it cool down and serve.

NUTRITIONAL INFORMATION:

Calories   150
Fat   13g
Carbohydrates   9g
Fiber   2g
Protein   3g
Sodium   110mg

Paleo Sweet Chocolate Drops

INGREDIENTS:

Optional Additions: Shredded Coconut, Chopped Nuts, Sea salt,
1/2 c. Coconut Oil
1/2 c. unsweetened Cocoa Powder
1/3 c. Honey

DIRECTIONS:

•Combine honey, coconut oil and cocoa powder in a food processor and process until you produce a smooth consistency.
•Spoon small mounds and place on the baking sheet or platter and place in the fridge or freezer to set.
•If you like to add more toppings, add it before placing them in the freezer.
•Keep them in an air tight container in your fridge or freezer.

NUTRITIONAL INFORMATION:

Calories   410
Fat   33g
Carbohydrates   33g
Fiber   5g
Protein   4g
Sodium   210mg

Complete Paleo Smoothie Recipe

INGREDIENTS:

½ c. frozen raspberries
1 avocado
1-2 tbsp. unsweetened cocoa powder
2 c. coconut milk

2 frozen bananas

DIRECTIONS:

•Peel off your bananas. If you will use frozen bananas, allow it to thaw for 10 mins. before peeling.
•Add all the ingredients in the blender and process well.
•Pour in a serving glass and enjoy.

NUTRITIONAL INFORMATION:

Calories   410
Fat   21g
Carbohydrates   51g
Fiber   15g
Protein   12g
Sodium   130mg

Paleo Berries And Watermelon Smoothie

INGREDIENTS:

1 c. fresh raspberries
1 c. frozen blueberries
1 c. ice
2 c. cubed watermelon

DIRECTIONS:

•In your blender, add all the ingredients and set at high-speed and pulse until smooth and creamy.
•Pour in a serving glass and serve.

NUTRITIONAL INFORMATION:

Calories   100
Fat   0.5g
Carbohydrates   26g

Fiber	6g
Protein	2g
Sodium	0mg

Peach-Coconut Paleo Smoothie

INGREDIENTS:

1 c. chilled full fat coconut milk
1 c. ice
2 large peeled and cut into chunks fresh peaches
Fresh lemon zest, to taste

DIRECTIONS:

•In your blender add coconut milk, peaches and ice. With the use of a microplane add some fresh lemon zest gratings.
•Set the blender at high speed and pulse until smooth and creamy.

NUTRITIONAL INFORMATION:

Calories	340
Fat	29g
Carbohydrates	23g
Fiber	6g
Protein	4g
Sodium	20mg

Cherry-Coconut Paleo Smoothie

INGREDIENTS:

1 c. coconut milk
1 c. pitted frozen cherries
1 tablespoon cacao powder
1 tablespoon MCT oil

DIRECTIONS:

•Place all the ingredients in a blender and process until smooth and creamy.

•Transfer in a serving glass and enjoy.

NUTRITIONAL INFORMATION:

Calories   230
Fat   18g
Carbohydrates   18g
Fiber   2g
Protein   2g
Sodium   10mg

Baked Squash Stuffed With Cranberry, Apple And Walnut

INGREDIENTS:

¼ teaspoon ground nutmeg
½ c. chopped walnuts
½ c. dried cranberries
1 halved and seeded acorn squash
1 tablespoon coconut oil
1 tablespoon ground cinnamon
2 to 3 chopped apples
3 tablespoon raw honey
Sea salt

DIRECTIONS:

•Pre-heat your oven to 400 degrees Fahrenheit.

•Rub 1 tablespoon of honey in the cut sides of the squash and season with ½ tablespoon of cinnamon.

•On a large baking sheet, place the squash and bake for 30 to 35 mins.

•Over medium-high heat, heat a skillet and melt the coconut oil.

•Add the walnuts, 1 tablespoon raw honey, nutmeg, apples, cinnamon, cranberries and a pinch of salt.
•Cook until the apples are tender or for 5 to 7 mins.
•Place the apple mixture into the squash.
•Return the stuffed squash in the oven and bake for another 10 to 15 mins. and serve.

NUTRITIONAL INFORMATION:

Calories	690
Fat	27g
Carbohydrates	118g
Fiber	16g
Protein	7g
Sodium	400mg

Paleo Choco-Sunflower Smoothie

INGREDIENTS:

1 1/2 c. Almond Milk, Unsweetened
1 teaspoon Cacao Powder
2 frozen Bananas
2 tablespoon Organic Sunflower Seed Butter, Unsweetened
4 pitted Medjool Dates

DIRECTIONS:

•Add all the ingredients in a high speed blender and process on high until smooth and creamy.
•Pour in a serving glass and serve.

NUTRITIONAL INFORMATION:

Calories	369.5
Fat	13g
Carbohydrates	70g
Fiber	0g

Protein	6.25g
Sodium	0mg

Healthy Paleo Lemon Cookies

INGREDIENTS:

1 1/2 teaspoon lemon extract
1 1/3 cup blanched almond flour
1 tablespoon lemon zest
1/2 teaspoon baking soda
1/3 cup maple syrup
1/4 cup refined melted coconut oil
1/8 teaspoon salt
2 tablespoon coconut flour

DIRECTIONS:

•Combine the maple syrup, lemon extract, coconut oil and lemon zest in a large mixing bowl.
•Add the coconut flour, salt, almond flour and baking soda. You will produce a thin and wet mixture and much more like a batter than dough.
•Chill the mixture to firm up the mixture. Allow the mixture to sit for 5 mins. and store it in the fridge for 30 mins. or until firm.
•Pre-heat your oven to 350 degrees Fahrenheit and use parchment paper to line the baking sheet.
•If you want bigger cookies, roll into six 50g balls. If you want it smaller, roll into nine 35g balls. Arrange them in the baking sheet 3 inches apart and press the bowls down using your palm.
•Bake for 12 minutes the smaller cookies and for 15 minutes the larger cookies or until the cookies are lightly browned. The cookies may slightly crack so don't worry.
•Once done take it out of the oven. Allow them to cool down on the pan completely.

•Keep them in an airtight container for up to four days.

Calories   200
Fat   14g
Carbohydrates   20g
Fiber   0g
Protein   3g
Sodium   250mg

Paleo Pumpkin Pie And Banana Smoothie

INGREDIENTS:

1 teaspoon Maple Syrup
1 1/2 frozen bananas
1/8 teaspoon Allspice
1/2 c. pumpkin puree
1/8 teaspoon Cinnamon (plus 1/8 tsp to garnish)
1 1/2 c. almond milk unsweetened
1/8 teaspoon Nutmeg
1/4 teaspoon Vanilla Extract
1/8 teaspoon Ginger

DIRECTIONS:

•Add all the ingredients in your blender, except for the cinnamon.
•Set your blender to high and blend until smooth and creamy.
•Pour smoothie in a tall glass and garnish it with cinnamon. Serve.

NUTRITIONAL INFORMATION:

Calories   160

Fat   2.5g
Carbohydrates   50.9g
Fiber   0g
Protein   3g
Sodium   0mg

Paleo Coconut-Pumpkin Smoothie

INGREDIENTS:

1 c. coconut milk
¼ c. organic pumpkin puree
2 tsp. pumpkin pie spice
1 frozen sliced banana
1 cup ice

DIRECTIONS:

•Add the pumpkin, banana, coconut milk, ice, and pumpkin pie spice into your blender.
•Blend on high speed until smooth and creamy.

NUTRITIONAL INFORMATION:

Calories   350
Fat   29g
Carbohydrates 24g
Fiber   5g
Protein   3g
Sodium   95mg

Conclusion

Thank you again for downloading this book!

I hope this book was able to help you to understand what paleo diet is and how effective it is.

The next step is to try out some of the recipes in this book and find out on your own how paleo diet can make you healthy and fit.

Thank you and good luck!

Part 2

Introduction:

The Hunter Vs The Hunted: Which One Do You Want to Be?

I'd like to introduce you to two different types- ancient man and modern man. Ancient man (and woman!) was a strong, healthy, alert hunter who was on top of the food chain. Modern man has lost the natural survival instincts and skills to be the sharp, fit and vigorous hunters that our ancient ancestors were. Instead modern man has become the hunted, a weak, sick, overweight and exhausted prey that is no longer a survivor. Let's take a look at how the hunted modern man compares to the ancient hunter. Modern man has a hard time waking up in the morning. He has to hit the snooze button a couple of times before he can finally manage to drag himself out of bed. He stands up unsteadily, feeling aches and pains in his joints, bones and muscles as he staggers into the bathroom. Once there, he might catch a glimpse of his reflection in the bathroom mirror and be unpleasantly surprised by what he sees: An exhausted expression, bleary eyes ringed with dark, unhealthy looking under eye circles, dull, lifeless looking skin and prematurely graying or receding hair and a bloated body that just keeps piling on the pounds no matter how hard he tries to eat healthy. If that's the reflection that also faced you in the mirror this morning, then you are like millions of other Americans who seem to be growing sick, fat, tired and older than their age, at breakneck speed. But what's behind this epidemic of illness and weight gain, you may be wondering. Let's take a look at the next step of modern man's morning routine for clues as to the most likely culprit.

At some point during the morning rush, modern man stops for a quick breakfast and grabs whatever is convenient. This usually means packaged, highly processed breakfast foods like frozen waffles, pop tarts or other "hearty" breakfast pastry goods with enough sugar in them to make him feel momentarily awake and energized. Then again, perhaps he will choose something more health conscious and opt for a better, more nutritionally balanced meal, like the kind promoted by the food pyramid: something like a bowl of "healthy" whole wheat cereal and some low-fat milk, a granola bar or a multi-grain bagel (without any butter), all washed down with a nice, tall glass of orange, or some other packaged fruit juice.

Modern man is often concerned about health and listens to the advice of conventional nutritionists and doctors, so he probably feels that he's done a great job choosing the second type of breakfast. In fact, as long as he steers clear of so-called dangerous foods like eggs, butter, fatty meats and keeps everything in his fridge, from yogurt to milk, strictly low-fat or fat-free, nutritionists, doctors and dieticians will tell him that he's eating a healthy diet and has nothing to worry about.

So if that's true, why does he feel so tired, even after that "energizing" breakfast? Why is it difficult for him to even climb into his car and drive to the office and why does he feel like he's run a marathon by the time he sits down at his desk? He's not alone there, either. This is why coffee has become the nation's number one fuel, helping people to get through hours of seated work. During his long workday, the few times he'll get up, other than bathroom breaks, will be in order to re-fill his mug of sugary coffee or stock up on some quick, high-calorie, processed snacks, because his "super-nutritious" breakfast and heavy lunch have actually left him feeling completely exhausted and wiped out.

By the time modern man's workday is over, he is thoroughly drained of all energy and can only drive home and collapse on the couch with a rushed fast-food dinner. He will probably stay on the computer or watch television late into the night and when he does finally climb into bed, he will most likely find it hard to get to sleep. The next morning, the poor quality of his sleep will catch up with him as he struggles to find the strength to roll out of bed all over again.

When it comes to health, modern man suffers all kinds of non-communicable diseases and conditions that ancient man has never heard of. Modern man is a victim of everything from diabetes to autoimmune disorders, different types of cancer and cardiovascular diseases to organ failure and dementia and is constantly being hunted by the rising risk of obesity, premature aging and depression. He spends a huge portion of his income on medical care and expensive prescription drugs but he only gets sicker, more tired, more overweight and unhealthier with every dollar he spends. Does this sound familiar?

If it does, that's because the routine I just described is extremely common nowadays. In fact, being weak, exhausted, ill and overweight has become the norm, not the exception for most people. But it wasn't always this way. Once, the average human was a lean, well-muscled, quick-thinking, agile and well-balanced survivor- at the top of the game and the food chain mentally, physically and emotionally. This kind of ancient human, let's call him the Hunter,(or the huntress, as the case may be) lived a totally different life than we do today and it is this lifestyle that is the secret to the Hunter's health, vigor and fitness. Let's take a look at how the Hunter's daily routine compares to the modern man's routine:

The Hunter was an early riser. As the sun came up, the Hunter would instinctively rise as well, because his body was still in tune with the natural rhythms of nature. He would spring up easily from the ground where he slept without having to struggle or fight off drowsiness. Because his health was at optimal levels, he was able to wake up alert, energetic and prepared to protect himself from any threats in his environment. The Hunter's morning routine did not include a large, carbohydrate-filled breakfast like ours often do today. Instead, he would have eaten(if he was hungry) a light, animal protein rich meal such as a handful of leftovers from the previous evening's dinner, drank from his store of clean, pure water and headed out into the wild, for a full day of outdoor activity. As a hunter, he would have

151

relied on his health, fitness and alertness every day to ensure his own survival and that of his family unit, meaning that he was typically responsible for bringing home vital food supplies.

Unlike the modern man who is a prisoner to an inactive desk job, the Hunter would therefore spend a large portion of his day stalking and hunting in the sun and fresh air. This would only increase his health and energy as he absorbed vital vitamin D from the sun's rays and got plenty of natural intermittent exercise from his stop-and-start movements. The Hunter was not tied to ridiculous and unnatural food rules like the ones we are taught by nutritionists and conventional doctors these days so he would eat sparingly throughout the day, neither over-snacking nor worrying about stuffing down large meals at precise times. Instead, he would listen to his own body for the cues that would tell him how much food he needed at any given time. The fatty, protein laden morning meal he had eaten earlier would help to nourish his brain and body, giving him a stable source of energy and the mental clarity needed to keep an eye on the animals he was seeking to hunt as well as avoiding threats and dangers like large carnivores, poisonous snakes and insects and dangerous terrain. Because the Hunter was not slowed down by excess weight or flagging energy like the modern man is today, he was able to survive and excel, no matter how challenging his environment was.

By the time the hunting day was done and he had captured his prey, he would still have all the energy required to drag his prize back home to the cooking fire. Unlike modern man, the Hunter lived in perfect harmony with the natural cycle of the day so once it was dark and he had eaten his meal of rich nourishing animal proteins and fats along with perhaps a handful of seeds or wild grown vegetables, he would begin to slip into a meditative, calm state, ready for a deeply revitalizing, healing sleep. As he slept, the Hunter didn't have to worry about being woken by a beeping cell phone or flashing lights from electronic gadgets like we do today. He was able to rest in total darkness, allowing his body to repair and restore every tissue and cell to perfect working order, preventing damage and disease and helping him to wake, ready to face any challenges the next day.

Modern man faces many challenges today, but most of them are within his power to change while our ancestor the Hunter was surrounded by many unpredictable challenges and dangers. Still, modern man is failing miserably at meeting his challenges while the Hunter successfully beat all of the odds and not only survived but THRIVED in his difficult environment. Modern man is a victim while ancient man was a victor. Modern man is HUNTED by illness, obesity, exhaustion and depression while ancient man was the ultimate HUNTER. Why? The answer is quite simply the Paleolithic lifestyle. Living in a Paleolithic (Paleo for short) way means the difference between being lean , healthy and active and being tired, ill and overweight,. It's the difference between having wonderful mental clarity and alertness or always feeling like your thinking is somehow cloudy and slow. Paleo is not just about weight loss. Yes, you will definitely lose any excess weight and easily attain the most balanced and physically fit body possible with this lifestyle but it provides benefits that go far beyond just that. In fact, Paleo living can do everything from improve your health, prevent diseases like type 2 diabetes, autoimmune disorders, cardiovascular and neurological diseases to heal and treat systemic candida infections, give your sharper thinking and reactions and even clear your skin.

Paleo is NOT a diet. It is a lifestyle shift that unleashes the inner hunter in you, providing you with the ability to naturally become the best, quickest, fittest, strongest and healthiest versions of ourselves that you can be. Paleo is NOT another fad-diet that pushes you to purchase a lot of expensive, low- nutrient, high-carb, sugary and chemical laden packaged "diet" foods. It is an amazingly powerful way of eating, drinking, exercising and being that WORKS because it is basically a step-by-step return to the healthy, fit and strong state humans used to exist in-and best of all, it doesn't have to be expensive. If you are looking for a way to completely transform your body, mind and energy levels but you're worried about investing in a lot of costly diet items and exercise gear, then Paleo is definitely for you! Paleo is all about using what's at hand to sharpen and hone your body and mind until you are at the peak of physical and mental fitness, just as our hunter-gatherers used what was available to them to become the ultimate survivors. If you've had enough of all of the conventional and misleading nutrition and fitness advice that has made modern humans so out of shape, overweight, exhausted and sick, if you're ready to bypass the expensive gimmicky diets that NEVER really work, if you want to see yourself transformed into the most elite, most skilled, strong, fit and healthy you possible-WITHOUT wasting time or money, then you are definitely ready for PALEO.

Let's get started!

Chapter 1: What Is Paleo?

The Paleo (Paleolithic) diet, also known as the caveman diet, is a way of eating that tries to match the ancestral eating habits of the human race as closely as possible, in order to improve health and maximize fitness. The paleo diet is based on the fact that while we may have learned many things since the end of our ancient hunting and gathering societies, proper nutrition is not one of them. While modern day humans are more sophisticated and technologically advanced (and better groomed!), our ancient ancestors definitely beat us in the health, nutrition and fitness categories. Our modern day diets are stuffed with harmful ingredients and our health, weight and brains are suffering under the strain of the "modern" diseases like obesity, cardiovascular diseases, high blood pressure, diabetes, autoimmune disorders and dementia. The Paleo diet's main foundation is built on foods that our ancient hunter-gatherer ancestors would have eaten, such as meats, eggs, fats, nuts, seeds, greens and berries while it excludes the often dangerous and unnecessary foods that our ancestors never ate but form a big part of our poor diets today, such as grains of all kinds, refined sugars, processed foods with unnatural chemicals, additives and industrial cooking oils. Because ancient humans never had access to such items and because, despite the time gap between them and us, modern humans' bodies are still made the same way, it stands to reason that the foods our ancestors never ate is food we shouldn't be eating either. On the other hand, the foods that cavemen ate in abundance are nourishing, energy and life-sustaining foods that we no longer eat in the quantities we should. And what are the results?

With every passing generation, the human body is becoming weaker, more broken down, less-muscled, less-balanced, more overweight and diseases-riddled. The human brain is being attacked on all sides by artificial stimulation, stress, chemicals and sugars, resulting in cloudy thinking, memory loss and even complete loss of cognitive abilities.

While our ancient ancestors could hunt large animals with only a spear, we are too weak to climb up a flight of stairs. While our ancient ancestors could comfortably walk many miles through rough terrain, bare foot, we can't even imagine going 2 blocks down the road without a car. Ancient hunter-gatherers could calculate the dangers in a situation at lightning speed, making quick, life-saving decisions at the drop of a pin but today, we are losing the gift of speedy thinking and have a hard time remembering even familiar names and numbers.

While our ancient ancestors ate to the full, deeply enjoying their protein and nutrient rich real food while staying slim, ultra-fit and healthy, we are constantly counting calories, feeling guilty about every bite we eat, trying diet after diet and still piling on stubborn pounds, no matter what we do! Which one sounds like a healthy, beneficial diet to you? In fact, if you dropped those ancient hunters into our modern environment today, they might struggle to get used to the fast-paced, high-stress way we live and have some difficulty getting understanding our technology but on the whole, with their well-nourished, fast-thinking minds and healthy, agile, disease-resistant bodies, they would adapt much better than the average overweight, under-nourished, ill and out of shape modern human would if dropped into the wilderness.

So at its root, Paleo is basically about making a choice between survival and extinction, thriving and failing, fitness, health and strength or flabbiness, illness and weakness. It's about turning the clock back on your fatigued, ailing and weight-saddled body and going from being the victim of modern foods, diseases and stress to being the victor.

The choice is yours. Which one do you want to be-the hunter or the hunted? If you choose to be the hunter, then rest assured that you've come to the right place. The Paleo way of eating was voted the most effective diet of all time by thousands of people who've tied it worldwide for a very good reason-it REALLY works. Not in a "lose 5 pounds, put 2 back on, kind-of-feel-better" sort of way. No, when I say it works, I mean it works in a "completely change your body, lose and keep off all excess weight, get fitter, faster, stronger, leaner, feel better than you've ever felt before" kind of way! If that sounds good to you, then there's nothing left to do but get started:

Paleo improves your well-being, health, body weight and fitness by allowing you to eat REAL foods and cutting out all of the ARTIFICIAL, non-nourishing, damaging food items your body was never meant to consume.

Let's look at what foods should make up the bulk of your Paleo meal plan:

- Vegetables

- Meats

- Fish

- Eggs

- Fruits

- Nuts

- Seeds

And the items that you should strictly avoid on your Paleo eating plan are:

- Sugar

- Grains

- Artificial flavors, colors and additives

- All processed foods and beverages

- Legumes

Because Paleo is not a "diet" in the gimmicky, "eat only one or two types of food for a month" sense, it does allow you a large scope for personal choices and preferences as long as you are truly listening to your body and honoring its reactions and sensitivities. That's why certain foods are left in a sort of "free zone", meaning you can choose whether to add them into your diet at all, eliminate them completely or limit their intake, depending on your own unique reaction and tolerance level: These foods include:

- Dairy products

- Certain starchy vegetables

So now that we've got the most basic components Paleo down, you may be thinking: Isn't this going to be really expensive? I can tell you right away that you DO NOT need to spend tons of money to eat a successful and effective Paleo meal plan. In fact, many people find that, when they cut out all of the unnecessary spending on harmful, unnatural and super-fattening packaged foods and drinks, they actually end up putting more away in the bank each month than they ever did before they went Paleo. Not to mention all of the money that is saved from unpleasant and unfruitful medical spending as a result of your new diet that eliminates and prevents a huge array of diseases and conditions. And when it comes to exercise, because the Paleo way of life is about natural movement and not pounding away on some machine for hours, you don't have to worry about needing to splash out on pricey gym memberships and fancy workout gear to lose weight. And that's why Paleo is such a popular lifestyle and what this book is really about: harnessing all of the benefits of weight loss, health, renewed energy, rejuvenated mind, body and appearance while at the same time finding and using awesome techniques that will save you money and time and

158

generally make this the best, easiest and most natural change you've ever made.

Taking care of your health getting the body you deserve and protecting your mind and physique from the ravages of aging should never be a choice between money and well-being, and with Paleo it's not! Instead, utilize the step-by-step, easy to use advice and information in this book to achieve the health and fitness you desire without wasting a single cent!

Chapter 2: Great Health Doesn't Have To Break The Bank: Affordable Ways To Go Paleo

The Paleo way of eating is quickly catching on like wildfire, because it provides undeniable results. But the one thing that stands between even more people joining this health movement and gaining the bodies, brains and lives they've always wanted is price.

Many people insist that eating Paleo has to be expensive. In fact, it's one of the biggest excuses a lot of people use to justify their unhealthy, carb and sugar-loaded, fast food lifestyle.

That's why I wrote this book. Because the truth is, there is absolutely NO reason why eating Paleo has to cost more than eating the Standard American Diet (SAD). Thousands of people have been shocked by the fact that they are actually SAVING money by eating Paleo. You may be shaking your head in disbelief right now but I promise you that once you've read this guide on eating Paleo on a budget, you will never believe that Paleo is too expensive again. Are you ready to learn the secrets of shedding those pounds and kicking illness and fatigue to the curb for good, without wasting any of your hard-earned cash? If so, read on. I promise, it'll be well-worth your time:

1. **Cut Out The Middle**: What do I mean by this? The next time you go into your local grocery store, take a moment to notice how the items are laid out. You will quickly realize that all of the real food such as the fruits, vegetables, meat and deli counter and the dairy areas are all lining the edge of the grocery store while the conventional, commercially prepared, highly processed junk "food" is given pride of place, right smack dab in the center of the store. In fact, this is why so many people struggle to shop smart and bring

160

home healthy items. These fattening and disease causing products are constantly calling to shoppers from their privileged position in the middle of the store, beckoning you to come and spend your precious dollars on a bunch of chemically enhanced, toxic boxes and bags that will only leave you fat, sick, tired and miserable. So what is the number one rule of Paleo supermarket shopping? CUT OUT THE MIDDLE! That's right, ignore all of those aisles upon aisles of strategically positioned poisons and head straight for the out perimeter. Make a beeline for the fresh produce section where you can load up on a lot of fresh vegetables and some fruits, then go and stock up on some protein in the meat and deli sections. If you are dairy tolerant, make sure you stop off and pick up some whole fat, grass-fed milk and butter as well as cartons of eggs and then go right to the checkout counter without giving those middle aisles a second glance. I guarantee you that when you hear how little your whole grocery cart of food costs, your jaw will hit the floor. Why? Simply because cutting out the entire middle of the supermarket and ONLY buying real foods means BIG savings. Think about it: How much do you think the average American spends on unhealthy junk foods ranging from sugary, carb-loaded cereal boxes to bags and bags of cookies, chips and other snack items, not to mention dessert items like cakes, packs of donuts, cartons of ice cream and what about beverages? Don't forget all of the cans, jugs and bottles of soft drinks, diet drinks, sports and energy drinks as well as supposedly "healthy" processed fruit juices that most people can't go a single day without. Now remove all of these items from your grocery list. It looks pretty short right? This is the main secret behind why insiders often joke that once you go Paleo, your wallet gets heavier while your body gets lighter!

2. **Eat In:** A lot of Paleo eaters do this anyway, even if they aren't necessarily trying to save money. The simple fact is

that it's way easier to create simple, flavorful and delicious Paleo dishes at home for yourself and your family than trying to explain to every waiter you meet that no, pasta is not grain-free or quizzing the chef about just how many chemicals went into his special sauce.

In short, you have to be in control of what goes into your body to truly be an effective Paleo eater. Restaurants may seem like a fast option but in the end they are actually just a fast route to weight gain and health problems. Now let's talk about the money:

A moderately priced meal in the average restaurant can cost up to 15 dollars and if you are eating out even once a day, that really adds up. In one month you would be shelling out $450 on eating out alone and $900 on eating out, if there are two of you! The same People who claim Paleo is too expensive to be done on a budget are the ones who eat out regularly and when you really think about it, wouldn't you rather feed your body and mind ultra-nourishing, fresh and real food while saving money than waste both money and your health by eating chemically-enhanced "dead" restaurant meals at expensive prices? Now, keep in in mind that just because you've gone Paleo, it doesn't necessarily mean that you CAN'T eat out once in a while. It just means that you have to be more careful with your food selections and choose a restaurant that is honest about its ingredients, so you can ensure that your health is well cared for, at the same time as you enjoy your meal. On the flip side, cook at home way more often and you will find that not only will you see your monthly grocery bill drop drastically but so will your weight. It's a simple fact that commercially prepared meals aren't going to be as cleanly and healthily prepared as your own home cooking, so if you really want to give your body a good shot at getting all of the benefits of going Paleo, limit your restaurant trips and start preparing the food your body really craves at home. If you're worried about learning to cook Paleo, don't be. Simply check out the recipe index at the back of this book for easy, delicious and nutritious Paleo meals you can make in no time flat!

3. **Learn the 80/20 Theory:** Many famous proponents of the Paleo way of eating and living have been doing this for years and while they absolutely love the amazing results of their ancestral lifestyles they also understand that thousands of years have passed since we were hunter-gatherers and the modern world is not going to be as Paleo friendly as the ancient one was. Do they let this stop them from getting all of the benefits of Paleo and enjoying themselves and their lives at the same time? No! In fact, that's where the 80/20 school of thought comes in. The 80/20 principle basically states that as long as you are giving the Paleo way of eating and living a real and committed try and you are staying away from the biggest dietary and lifestyle offenders, you don't have to stress unnecessarily about the one or two times that modern life has made it difficult or impossible to make the most Paleo choice. For example, what do you do if you have to eat in a restaurant and the grass-fed beef option is too expensve? Simple, you just choose another protein and animal fat rich option like non-grass fed steak or chicken, remove any non-Paleo side dishes and sauces and ENJOY your meal!

Paleo is not about trying to go back thousands of years in the past. That would be impossible and some would say, rather unpleasant, no matter how much money you spend. Instead, it is about harnessing the ancient secrets of eating and living that made hunter-gatherers so much healthier than modern man and using that information as a way to get and stay healthy and fit in today's world. 80/20 basically means that if you're sticking fully to Paleo 80% of the time, then you will see amazing results and get all of the benefits, regardless of the 20% where life happens and you can't always make the best Paleo choice. This theory has helped thousands of people get and stay Paleo because it allows for people with different budgets and different schedules to all get what they need out of Paleo. It's not hard and fast rule, so for instance, you may be able to do 90%perfect Paleo and only have to make compromises 10% of the time. In that case, you're doing great and will see results a little faster but those that are 80/20 will also be getting excellent and life-changing results too. That's the great thing about the Paleo way of eating and living. It really is a lifestyle instead of a fad diet. Paleo doesn't tell you that you have to live off of expensive food like asparagus and lobster, it doesn't mean you have to buy fancy vitamins, supplements and weight loss shakes. It quite simply means living as closely to your body's natural, ancestral way of being as possible. And guess what? Whether you are doing 80/20 or 90/10 or 100%, Paleo really works. It delivers jaw-dropping results in a short amount of time and as long as you don't go back to sugary, carb-loaded, processed eating, you will continue to see those results for the REST OF YOUR LIFE! Let's be clear about a few things though: 80/20 doesn't mean eating perfectly Paleo 80 percent of the time and gorging on sugary, carb-loaded or chemical packed foods and beverages for the remaining 20 percent.

It means that after eating perfectly Paleo 80 percent of the time, if your budget and time constraints make the remaining 20 percent difficult to get perfect, you choose the next, most-Paleo option available to you. So if you eat free-range eggs most of the time, but this week you can only afford regular eggs, it doesn't mean that you reach for a bagel or cereal instead. It means that you get the regular eggs and maybe you add a dollop of grass-fed butter to them for an extra, more Paleo boost.

So, if sometimes you have to choose less-expensive and slightly less-Paleo options to make Paleo living work for you and your budget, don't sweat it. Doing Paleo 80/20 is literally a million times better than eating the standard American diet so many people are addicted to or even one of these low-fat, high-carb fad diets that doctors and nutritionists swear by. If you can manage 80/20 then be very proud of yourself, you WILL see the results your body and brain deserve.

4. **Learn to Shop Paleo:** While simply cutting out all of the overpriced, manufactured processed junk that makes up the bulk of modern man's diet is enough to slice down your grocery bill, knowing how to shop for the right ingredients will make your Paleo meal plan a successful, delicious and inexpensive cinch!

Get Your Staples: As you know by now, the Paleo way of eating is grain-free but that doesn't mean that our ancient hunter ancestors lived off of just meat, meat and more meat. When it comes to Paleo staple, nutritious vegetables are the way to go, and the best part is that they are the cheapest items in your grocery store! Grab a whole bunch of leafy greens to round out your protein portions and you'll be shocked to see just how little you actually spend.

Head to the Great Outdoors: No, I don't mean you should go looking for food in the wilderness. I just mean that you should try your local outdoor farmer's market for the freshest, least expensive and most delectable array of fresh produce around. Farmer's markets are THE secret to shopping Paleo on a budget and getting the very best, most nutritious food possible.

Don't Sweat the Small Stuff: As you begin your Paleo journey, don't let the idea of shelling out big bucks for organic, naturally cultivated foods scare you off. While eating organic foods is definitely a great and healthy way to make sure we are living as closely to our ancient eating patterns as possible, it is not the be-all and end-all of the Paleo eating plan. If organic is too expensive for the majority of your meals, don't stress yourself out too much. Some organic produce is more important than other types. Steer clear of the most pesticide soaked types of produce(this can vary by area) and the crops most likely to be GMO and when it comes to the rest, just make sure that you are getting ample amounts of Paleo-friendly fruits and veggies and don't worry about focusing on just organic for the meantime. It is important to really get into Paleo-eating and allow your body to show you how much it truly needed this life change. After that, you can choose for yourself how much you're willing to spend on organic and grass-fed food products. And make no mistake, even if you aren't eating all organic, non-GMO and grass-fed items, as long as what you're eating is Paleo, you're doing a whole lot more for your body than somebody regularly consuming grains and sugars(no matter how organic they may be).

Store Up Your Prey: Despite being called "uncivilized" societies, did you know that hunter-gatherers never wasted food like we do and were very clever at finding ingenious ways to preserve their food supplies to last them through lean times and harsh winters? With methods like fermenting and burying food, these hunters were able to keep their families and themselves fed and healthy to survive and thrive another year. Paleo eating is sustainable eating. How can you apply this to your own life? Well, don't worry, I'm not asking you to dig a hole in your backyard and ferment your freshly bought salmon steaks! What I mean by storing is making sure that you're thinking longer term rather than just "what should we have for dinner tonight?" This is where a lot of modern people go wrong today. We tend to think about food when we get hungry instead of planning ahead. When you look at your food as supplies and provisions that are there to feed AND nourish your healthy lifestyle, you'll stop wanting to reach for something fast, full of calories and "easy" and instead, map out a delicious plan to stay fit, slim and satisfied. Make a strategy and a budget and stick to it. Buy more pricey items like grass-fed beef and cage-free poultry meat in bulk and freeze them in individual labelled bags so that they can last for many months. When you need to get a quick meal together, it is as easy as grabbing an individual bag out of the freezer and defrosting! If you have other Paleo friends (we are a large community) consider buying in bulk together for truly HUGE savings. Make sure you store all of your fruits and vegetables properly, wrapping them in clean paper or cloth to keep them from getting frostbitten or wilted in your veggie section. Never waste leftovers. Simply store them well and use them for the next day's breakfast. Trust me, once you learn to store like a hunter, you'll find it easy to keep your monthly grocery bill well into the very low hundreds!

Make Smart Paleo Swaps: When people say Paleo food is expensive, it's because they think that a high protein, animal fat diet must be all fillet mignon and exotic fruits. That is simply not the case. There are literally tons of very smart Paleo swaps that you can make that will quickly cut down the cost and still deliver great Paleo nutrition and intense, amazing flavor.

Eggs: If you're looking for high-quality protein that delivers a nutritious, filling, versatile and tasty meal, look no further than that carton of eggs in the dairy section! When you think about it, a dozen eggs rarely costs more than a couple of bucks and yet you can make everything from Paleo omelets and scrambles to really gourmet fare like a no-crust, vegetable quiche or a cheesy, delicate French soufflé, just by cracking a couple!

Meat: When it comes to meat, don't feel that it has to be steak all the time. Instead, swap that steak for a delicious ground beef patty, cooked to perfection and garnished with full-fat butter. Also, don't let yourself be limited to the meat selection at your grocery store. Get to know your local butcher well and you will find that you can buy high-quality cuts for much less than in the supermarket when you purchase directly from the source.

Poultry: Eat the savory and nutrition-packed dark meat. Seriously, although white, lean chicken breast has gained a reputation as the "health" food of choice among the low-fat crowd, that's not what Paleo advocates. Eat the fattier, more flavorful dark meat for a fantastic source of rich nutrition and taste that will slim you down and bulk up your wallet at the same time!

Vegetables: Pre-washed, peeled and chopped veggies can be much more costly than whole ones at any grocery store. The answer: Do it yourself! Spending a few extra minutes washing, peeling and dicing your own vegetables at home will save you money and guarantee you the freshest, cleanest veggies possible. Also, keep in mind that vegetables lose their nutrients quickly after being exposed to air so those store bought ones may potentially have far less vitamins and minerals than the ones you prep at home.

Fruits: Always buying the freshest, most exotic fruits can get quite pricey. Instead, aim for making up a part of your fruit intake with delicious and healthy smoothies and sorbets made from whole, frozen berries. They are still packed with vitamins and nutrients and make for a budget-easy way to get the fruit you crave.

5. **Think Long Term:** Sure, grabbing a fast-food burger may seem like a simple, easy and cheap way to fill up for the moment, but if you look beyond the moment, you know that it has far-reaching and very expensive consequences. Food can be your medicine or it can be your poison, it can be your body's best friend or its very worst nightmare. The choice is yours. SO when you think about saving a couple of bucks and a few minutes of prep time by just ordering takeout or something quick from a drive-thru, don't forget that your body is being seriously damaged by each and every single poor eating choice you make and that one day, sooner rather than later, you will have to deal with the consequences. The consequences usually come in the form of a surprise injury or sudden illness, bringing with t huge medical bills or even just overall exhaustion, major weight gain and fatigue, making it impossible to do your job or live your life to the fullest. Don't forget that the average hospital stay can easily average up to $20,000. That's 20,000 dollars for ONE single stay, because of ONE easily preventable health issue that the Paleo way of eating can help to eliminate! So when someone tells you that Paleo is expensive, remember that they are speaking from a place of inexperience: They either

don't know or haven't learned how Paleo can be eaten on a budget and how it can help to prevent and heal so many costly medical issues and restore your energy, youthful vibrancy, health and appetite for life. How much is your health worth?

.

The Paleo way of eating and living can completely transform your health and life and the truth is that it doesn't have to cost more than sustaining an unhealthy fast-food habit or guzzling gallons of soft drinks. This book is packed with ideas and information that will help you to make your Paleo journey an easy, budget-friendly and delicious path for healing, rejuvenation, weight loss and longevity!

In the next chapter, we'll look at the one most important item you MUST stop poisoning your body and brain with right away!

Chapter 3: The Bitter Secret About A Sweet Poison That Is Ruining Your Health!

Our ancient ancestor, the Hunter, lived a hard life. Without a constant supply of food, adequate shelter or any medical care to speak of, he faced many challenges in trying to stay alive. And yet, even though we have plenty of food, housing and medical care, modern humans are facing a threat that is just as deadly if not deadlier than the ones faced by the Hunter. This threat is called sugar and it is literally killing millions of people around the world. You may think I am over-emphasizing the risk but consider this: Even as you read these words, sugar is busily causing terrifying and painful life-threatening conditions like metabolic syndrome, obesity, type 2 diabetes, cardiovascular diseases, strokes, autoimmune diseases from MS to lupus and neurodegenerative diseases like Parkinson's and Alzheimer's Disease. It is no wonder that sugar is now recognized by leading doctors and researchers as the single most deadly killer of our time. According to Dr. Robert Lustig, a renowned endocrinologist who has studied the link between sugar and ill-health, up to a whopping 75 % of all diseases afflicting Americans are now brought on by the SAD (Standard American Diet) that sugar plays such a huge part in.

This means that the tens of millions of people who are suffering from the myriad of diseases brought on by consuming sugar are actually suffering needlessly! That's right. These conditions and diseases are completely preventable. How, you ask? The answer to that is very, very simple: Put down this book for a moment and walk over to your fridge and cupboards. Now, get rid of every last item containing refined sugar, from that big bag of cane sugar to all of those sodas, snacks, cereals and even canned goods, packed chockfull of sugar, dextrose, maltose, high fructose corn syrup and all of the other guises sugar hides its deadly poison in.

It really is that easy. If you do nothing else that is advised in this book to change your life and save yourself from the tidal wave of obesity, failing health and lethal diseases, taking this one simple action will SAVE YOUR LIFE! That's a big claim, but don't take my word for it. Take a look at the shocking evidence that backs up my statement, below:

Sugar and Diabetes: In a recent study, scientists looked at populations living in 17 different countries around the globe over a period of 10 years, in order to see whether different foods like meats, oils, fibers and sugar as well as social and economic factors like poverty, geography and aging had any kind of impact on the prevalence of type 2 diabetes. What these researchers found shocked everybody No type of food or socioeconomic factor had any kind of impact on the development of type 2 diabetes, except for one: Sugar. Out of all factors, only sugar availability was directly linked to the rapid rise of type 2 diabetes in populations around the world! This is as close as the medical and scientific world has ever come to admitting that yes, sugar consumption does lead to type 2 diabetes.

Sugar, High Fructose Corny Syrup and High Cholesterol: Several groundbreaking studies have shown a clear association between consumption of sugars like high fructose corn syrup and having higher levels of (bad) LDL cholesterol. These studies have shown that not only do your LDL levels go up when you consume sugar, but your risk of developing a variety of life-threatening cardiovascular diseases also goes up. I'm pretty sure that suddenly those helpings of sugar in your coffee cup aren't looking quite as enjoyable anymore.

Sugar Calories and Obesity: It has also been proven that all calories are not the same. When test subjects were made to replace nearly 30% of their daily total calories with calories from sugar-laden drinks, their weight shot right up, even though they were consuming the same amount of calories as usual. Nothing had changed except where their calories were coming from. What does this tell us? Calories from sugar are able to promote rapid weight gain, lead to obesity and even clog your heart's arteries in a way that non-sugar calories simply do not.

Sugar and Metabolic Syndrome: Metabolic syndrome, a collection of related diseases like type 2 diabetes, high blood pressure, high cholesterol with poor LDL to HDL balance, cardiovascular disease, non-alcoholic liver damage, a variety of cancers and dementias, is making major health headlines these days, as a newly emerging and dangerous threat. But if you thought this condition affected only overweight people, think again. Data now shows us that at least 40% of all normal weight people in the United States have developed one or all of the diseases and disorders that make up the metabolic syndrome spectrum. At the same time, a frightening 80% of all obese people manifest these diseases, too! This makes metabolic syndrome the most serious health emergency facing mankind today. So just what is behind its scary rise? That's right, sugar! Studies have proved that added sugars in foods and beverages are directly to blame for liver-contaminating, life-span shortening effects of this deadly syndrome! If you want to make sure that your body does not become yet another victim or statistic of this fast rising disease, kick sugar out of your life for good!

Sugar and Ageing: If you're like a lot of people, you have several expensive lotions and skin creams lining your bathroom shelves, in order to slow down or prevent the ageing process. But I've got news for you. If you are regularly consuming sugar in your food and beverages, then those lotions and creams won't do you an ounce of good. The reason I say this is because it is a fact that sugar consumption rapidly speeds up the ageing process, leaving you looking and feeling tired, ill and far older than your real age. It does this by acting on your proteins, lipids and your DNA to create permanent damage by literally binding fructose to them.

Your skin becomes hard, rough, inflexible and dull. Instead of bouncing, it sags. Instead of lifting, it droops and quickly forms unsightly wrinkles. On the flip-side, try going without sugar for just a few days and then take a look in the mirror. The sudden health, glow and vitality of your complexion will do far more to convince you that you can put a stop to premature ageing by ditching the toxic white stuff, than all of the research in the world!

Sugar and Your Brain: "Sugar will rot your brain." How many times did you hear those words while growing up? Well, the facts are in and it is absolutely true. Even though it is impossible to say exactly how healthy the ancient brains of hunter-gatherers were, we do know that neurodegenerative diseases such as Parkinson's and Alzheimer's are not a "natural Part of ageing" as we are so often led to believe. We know this because, even though these diseases are highly common now in the WEST, they aren't in the rest of the world. If you look at other nations around the globe, you will find that actually, neurodegenerative disease and cognitive decline are very rare. On the other hand, here in the US and the West in general, rates of these neurodegenerative diseases are quickly skyrocketing, with even people as young as in their thirties presenting with signs of early onset dementia, for the first time ever in human history!

Why is this case? Well, if you look at the diets of developing nations where sugar is rarely eaten or drunk, you will quickly see that they also have correspondingly low rates of incidence for cognitive decline and dementias of any kind. When you look at the Western diet, however (especially the Standard American Diet), you can clearly see that it has been built on a dangerous foundation of added sugars. At the same time, you'll also notice that rates of cognitive decline and dementias of ALL kinds are rising right through the roof. This is not merely a hypothesis. Research shows us that consuming sugar leads to the disruption of your insulin levels. This then leads to a severe buildup of highly damaging amyloid proteins in your brai. Amyloid proteins are responsible for the development of dementia. Other studies also show that older people who ate diets that contained more sugars were much more likely to develop Alzheimer's or Parkinson's disease.

Anecdotally, people who go on the Paleo eating plan for the first time often report that removing sugar from their lives dramatically improves their long and short-term memory, their thinking skills, reaction time and ability to focus fully while carrying out difficult tasks. When we look at the lifestyles of our hunter-gatherer ancestors this makes perfect sense. The Hunter was never at risk of these mind-ruining and deadly diseases because he never had refined sugar available to him. Honey, his main source of sweetness, was a rare and very precious treat that was fiercely guarded by bees and therefore, not an easy, every day snack or staple, as so many sugary items have become for us today. As a result, the Hunter was able to stay sharp, alert and ultra-responsive to any changing circumstances or threats in his environment, allowing him to live to see another day in the dangerous wilderness that he roamed through. These days, as modern humans, we also face numerous dangers and challenges to our survival and it is absolutely certain that consuming sugar places a real drag on our mental processes today and may completely rob us of our ability to think at all tomorrow, if we continue to consume it.

Sugar and Cancer: Famed Nobel Laureate in medicine, Otto Warburg Ph.D., found out long ago that sugar is cancer's favorite food of choice. He showed how cancer cells were completely different from our healthy cells when it came to sources they used for energy. Cancer always rely on glucose(sugar) to feed them and guarantee their survival and high sugar consumption nourishes theses diseased cells, allowing them to spread, multiply and eventually, kill.

Sugar has been proven to be a major contributor to the increasing incidence of breast cancer in countries where a

Western diet is widely consumed. Sugar has also been linked to a doubled and sometimes even tripled risk for pancreatic cancer, cancer of the biliary tract and liver cancer, among others. Starving cancer cells of their most loved food, sugar, can effectively force them to die off, because they cannot efficiently use any other food source for energy.

This list may seem frightening but the truth is, the diseases and disorders listed above are just a small sample of the many, many conditions that are caused by or exacerbated by sugar consumption. If you are convinced of sugar's deadly powers and you are ready to set yourself free from its addictive and destructive hold on you, checkout the list of items to eliminate and start you Paleo, sugar-free lifestyle today. You'll be saving your body, your brain and your life!

Remove The Following Sugars and Sugar Sources Completely from Your Diet:

- Table sugar

- All items containing added sugar, sucrose

- Anything containing:

- Sucrose

- Maltose

- Dextrose

- Dextran

- Dextrin

- Maltodextrin

- Fructose(Added)

- Glucose

- Galactose

- Lactose(Added)

- High Fructose Corn Syrup

- Glucose Solids

- Cane Juice

- Cane Juice Crystals

- Cane Juice (Dehydrated)

- Brown Sugar

- Barley malt

- Beet Sugar

- Corn Syrup

- Corn Syrup Solids

- Carob

- Malt Syrup

- Caramel

- Golden Syrup

- Turbinado Sugar

- Sorghum Syrup

- Diastase

- Ethyl Maltol

- Yellow Sugar

- Manitol

- Xylitol

Get rid of all packaged, processed foods (most of them are simply loaded with sugar) and all commercially prepared desserts, snacks and breakfast items. Make your own fresh sauces and condiments and do away with any store-bought ones because they are often a hidden sugar trap.

If you're wondering what you CAN use to add a little natural and healthy sweetness to your life, don't despair. There are some very good and completely natural, Paleo sweeteners out there that you can enjoy as part of an end of the week treat or a rare celebration:

Here is the list of fantastic tasting, natural, Paleo sweeteners to use once in a while:

- Organic Locally Sourced Raw Honey

- Pure Green Leaf Stevia or Pure Extract

- Dates(Especially Medjool Dates)

- Coconut Nectar

- Fruit juice (only fresh squeezed, real, organic

These five items are available in the wild and our hunter-gatherer ancestors could have accessed them sparingly, making these five sweeteners Paleo and perfectly OK for once in a while use.

Natural but Not as Fully Available In the Wild- Use Small Amounts Once in a Very Rare While

- Coconut sugar/crystals

- Maple syrup

- Palm sugar

These Sweeteners are Completely Artificial, Not Paleo and are Dangerous to Your Health, Never Use Them:

- **Aspartame (**Nutra-Sweet, Equal**)**

- Sucralose (**Spenda**)

- Tagatose (**PreSweet**

- Acesulfame K (**Sweet One**

- Stevia - white/bleached (**Truvia, Sun Crystals**)

- **Saccarin (**Sweet'N Low**)**

(If you're looking for more information on artificial sweeteners, make sure to check out the chapter on artificial additives and processed foods!)

Now that we've gotten this deadly "legal poison" out of the way, join me in the next chapter to find out why everyone is going against the grain and what this important Paleo move can do for your health, weight and energy!
See you there!

Chapter 4: All Grains A Strain On The Brain. Why Paleo Means Never Going Back To Grains!

If you are one of the millions of people who have been conscientiously following the "healthy eating" guidelines set out in the food pyramid and countless weight loss diets, by so-called experts, then you have probably struggling to understand why you are still experiencing bloating, exhaustion, unexplained and persistent weight gain as well as a general overall feeling of not being "well". Your fridge may be stocked with loads of heart-healthy, multi-grain, whole wheat foods and yet your cholesterol levels aren't looking very good and your low-fat, high grain diet seems not to be enough to keep your body from piling on the pounds. If this sounds familiar, then you are probably also disappointed, disillusioned and full of doubt when it comes to following yet another "diet". Well, don't despair because, as you will see, the Paleo way of eating is not simply another diet plan. It is a completely revolutionary way of resetting your body's clock to recapture the health, vigor, fitness, fat-burning and metabolism that human beings always naturally had. And in order to gain these amazing benefits, you have to do one very important thing: Ignore the experts! Yes, I said it! The USDA, the food pyramid, the doctors, nutritionists and the "diet gurus" everywhere who are trying to force you to deny your body's truth and instead, brainwash you into believing that eating a recommended 6-11 daily servings of something absolutely detrimental to human health is actually something good for you-ignore them all!

It may seem surprising to you that, when it comes to grains, the Paleo way of eating goes against the conventional advice of doctors and nutritionists but think about it: How many millions of people (yourself included) have tried to eat all of the grains prescribed as healthy by these same doctors and nutritionists?

179

And how many of those millions of people end up feeling sicker and more tired, looking older and more bloated, and suffering with everything from obesity to depression, autoimmune disorders to dementia? So when it come s to your own life, you've got to take back control and refuse to let the outdated and completely misleading nutritional guidelines of the food pyramid and the nutritionists lead you to physical and emotional pain, exhaustion and the total destruction of your mind and body. To win back your valuable health, you've got to go against the grain!

List of Grains to Eliminate From Your Diet:

- **Amaranth**

- **Barley**

- **Brown rice**

- **Brown rice bread**

- **Brown rice tortilla**

- **Buckwheat**

- **Kamut**

- **Bulgur**

- **Farro**

- **Emmer**

- **Einkorn**

- **Flaxseed**

- **Millet**

- **Oats**

- Oat bread

- Oatmeal

- Popcorn

- Whole wheat cereal

- Muesli

- Rolled oats

- Quinoa(not a "real" grain but nonetheless, a non-Paleo grain-like substance)

- Rye (Whole or Not)

- Sorghum

- Spelt

- Teff

- Triticale

- Wheat berries

- Whole grain cornmeal

You may be wondering, just what it is about grains that can cause such damage to the human body and brain Well, because grains affect us negatively on so many levels , there are many answers to that question. Let's look at some of them:

Diseases: We have been told for a very long time by scientists that disease is coded into human DNA and that our genes are the number one decider of whether we will get sick or not and what kind of diseases we may develop in the future. That simply is not true. Diseases are not inscribed in our destiny. Instead, it is our lifestyle choices that are the deciding factors between health and illness. Where do grains fit in to all of this? Grains cause diseases like gasoline fuels fires. We may eat them for many years without ever really realizing how we are dragging our bodies and minds to the very edge of destruction and then one day, when we tip over the edge, suddenly we find our health going up in flames.

Here are some of the top ways that grain consumption can totally throw off our bodies' natural balance, health and metabolism:

Grains Equal a Dangerous Carbohydrate Rush: Refined sugars aren't the only substance s we should be worried about. When it comes to triggering a speedy rise in our insulin levels, grains can be just as bad. Because grains are simple sugars, they are very rapidly and easily broken down into sugar. The resulting rise in our blood glucose levels signals the start of a crazy insulin rollercoaster in our bodies' that can leave us with permanent nerve, tissue and organ damage. When we eat the "recommended" diet of heaps upon heaps of grains, we often feel completely bone tired.

That is because all of those grains are taking their toll on our insulin levels, keeping them impossibly high for longer and longer periods, creating a truly frightening situation for our bodies and brains. Modern man is now facing an unprecedented epidemic of frequently elevated insulin levels. Normally, this hormone's primary job is to manage levels of sugar in your blood. When glucose levels stay too elevated for too long, the body is faced with an onslaught and as a result, develop a resistance to insulin. At this stage, even more insulin is produced in order to flood your cells with and the insulin rush plus insulin resistance pattern begins to emerge. When this happens metabolic syndrome, a syndrome with massive implications for the future health of mankind, begins to take place.

Constantly elevated levels of insulin are standing in the way of most Americans desire to lose weight because high insulin levels prevent the body from being able to burn off the fat, instead turning the body's attention to making the surplus of glucose in the blood into your main energy source. Whatever is left unused at the end of this process is quickly packed away on your body as stubborn fat. This stubborn fat then rapidly turns into a particularly difficult to lose store of stomach blubber and as we all know, those excessive tires of abdominal fat, called visceral fat, are the single most serious health threat of our time, bringing us face to face with the risk of heart attacks and strokes, aneurysms, type 2 diabetes –led organ death, vicious inflammation and breathing disorders such as emphysema. This is why we say those friendly USDA guidelines regarding the wonderful benefits of grains are some of the most deadly pieces of health advice you can take.

Aside from an insane carbohydrate load, grains also saddle the human digestive system with another very serious problem, anti-nutrients.

Phytates: Phytates are found in grains and their damaging effect on the human body comes from the way they bind themselves to the minerals such as calcium, iron, zinc, magnesium and copper in our food, preventing us from being able to absorb and utilize these minerals for our health and well-being. Even when eating a diet that is very rich in mineral content, you can end up with severe nutritional deficiencies. This makes those nutritional arguments that you should eat plenty of grains for their "healthy mineral content" completely pointless, because every time you eat a supposedly mineral-rich slice of whole wheat bread for instance, the phytates contained in that bread have basically stolen your desired mineral supply from you. A Paleo diet that is full of proteins, fats, vegetables, seeds, fruits and nuts can provide you with nutrients you can EASILY and FULLY use, unlike grain-based diets that strip away their "benefits" before you even get a chance to absorb them! (Note: Phytates are also found in much lower and less harmful amounts in nuts and seeds which are Paleo approved. To enjoy your nuts and seeds and still harness all of the nutrition you need, try soaking them in either water, a lemon and water mix or pure yogurt. This will "digest" the phytates for you so that your body doesn't have to do the hard work.

Lectins: Lectins are found in all grains and are extremely dense, tough and tiny, making them an absolute nightmare for the human digestive system. Leptins destroy the intestinal walls by allowing openings to be made in them and thus, allowing for the development of leaky gut disorder. They damage the gut lining which leads to leaky gut and other disorders. When leaky gut syndrome strikes, you know that autoimmune diseases and disorders are not far behind, as these openings in the intestinal wall lining can only mean that potentially toxic, undigested foods, bacteria and other harmful materials can easily slip out of the intestines through these holes, entering your blood and crossing the blood/brain barrier and without further ado, you can find yourself in a scary autoimmune cycle, facing down your own immune system and hoping that you will not destroy your own body. Lectins are impossible to destroy with heat so even if you cook them thoroughly, they will still remain tough and inedible. In addition to all of this, lectin actually suppresses your appetite control system, leaving you always feeling ravenous, constantly snacking and never full! Also, all members of the grass family contain very high amounts of lectin so it is very important to steer clear of wheats, wheat grass and other grass grains in particular. When our bodies come into contact with lectins, after a few run-ins, our immune systems react with ferocity, fighting by creating powerful antibodies to target and neutralize the foreign threat. However, what happens when your own tissue looks so similar to the lectins your body is fighting? The result is usually the large scale destruction of your own tissue, with your immune system going rogue and leaving you damaged, ailing and perhaps even in danger of losing organ function.

Gluten: Now for the third and perhaps, the very worst of the deadly grain quartet, gluten. Gluten is a difficult to breakdown protein that can be found in many commonly eaten grains such as:

- White Flour
- Whole Wheat Flour
- Durum Wheat
- Semolina
- Spelt
- Wheat Germ
- Wheat Bran
- Graham Flour
- Triticale
- Kamut

Gluten is commonly found in these food items as well:

- Cereal
- Crackers
- Sodas
- Beer
- Oats (see the section on oats below)
- Gravy
- Dressings
- Sauces
- Couscous
- Bread
- Flour Tortillas
- Pasta
- Cakes
- Muffins
- Pastries

Gluten is now found in much higher amounts within today's modern grains, with levels reaching 80 %, than ever existed in ancient grains. All gluten containing substances are capable of creating a state called agglutination, a reaction that causes suspended particles to coagulate in big clumps. What does this do to our bodies?

- Gluten-led agglutination causes the creation of pro-inflammatory chemicals, in response to what the body perceives as a major injury.
- Gluten destroys the protective covering over neurons, and stops nerve growth factor from helping neurons to live.
- Gluten acts on the body and brain like any viruses and research shows that the body views it as just such a dangerous invader, triggering a damaging response.
- Gluten forces the clumping of blood platelets, disrupting their normal functions.

The gliadin content in today's wheat also causes inflammatory cytokine activity that leads to numerous tiny holes being drilled into the important intestinal wall lining, resulting in a nasty case of leaky got (gut permeability). Zonulin, a protein molecule produced when we eat gluten, also contributes to leaky gut by loosening the usually tight junctions within the intestinal cell walls. This permeability opens up the gut, allowing undigested, partially digested and toxic food and other particles, like bacteria to slip into the bloodstream where they cause havoc. This in turn leads to diseases and disorders such as autoimmune disorders like chronic fatigue syndrome, rheumatoid arthritis, multiple sclerosis, lupus, chronic fatigue syndrome, fibromyalgia, inflammatory bowel disease (ulcerative colitis) and asthma. Up to a third of the adult population has lab visible amounts of anti-gliadin within their stools.

All Grains a Strain on Your Brain!

These anti-gliadin antibodies are the result of your body's protective response to the "invader" gluten and are a clear indication of inflammation. In the same way as it causes leaky gut, gluten can also cause leaky brain syndrome or increased permeability of the vital blood brain barrier. When gluten inflames the brain, it forces openings in what is a usually closed barrier, allowing numerous harmful food antigens and even bacterial pathogens to flood into the brain, causing disease, loss of cognitive abilities, loss of memory, anger, depression, confusion, and even certain manifestations of mental illness. The symptoms of brain fog and emotional disturbance are only sign posts, signaling that the constant inflammation your brain is being subjected to through gluten or grain consumption will eventually lead to a terrifying and painful neurodegenerative disease like Parkinson's , Alzheimer's disease or dementia. All grains effectively light your brain on fire and let it slowly burn its way down to the very end, causing untold suffering and much invisible damage before the results are clear. If that sounds scary, it's because it is. Our brains are our most important organs and safeguarding them has to be a priority for the survival minded human. Without a well- protected and well-functioning brain, you quickly go from being the predator to being the prey!

Protease Inhibitors: Aside from the gluten, lectin, phytates and elevated insulin response, grains also contain yet another dangerous stumbling block that trips up anybody trying to find the road to good health by including them into their diet. These stumbling blocks are protease inhibitors and they are the body's equivalent of gasoline being poured on a raging wildfire! When you consume grains of any kind, protease inhibitors slow down or stop proper digestion of protein within your gut. Not only does this mean you have an even harder time dealing with lectins, but it also means you can't digest those very beneficial proteins you're getting from nutrient rich sources. This basically boils down to one sad fact: It doesn't matter how much high quality, fantastic protein you're gulping down, protease inhibitors will not allow you to use them. So if you are eating rains, you may just as well NOT spend your money on buying expensive lean chicken breast, organic lamb meat or pastured beef, because in the end. Your body doesn't see an ounce of the benefits, so long as protease inhibitors are doing their dastardly work.

Paleo Alternatives to Grains: How to Make You No- Grain Diet Work For Your Body and Your Budget!

Just because you've gone Paleo does not mean you've suddenly become immune to the once in a rare while cravings for certain baked products. But when you're faced with that craving, does this automatically mean you should just go for the cake, cookies or pizza in front of you? Absolutely not, especially when there are some very Paleo ways to circumvent those cravings and still stay on track, healthy and happy. Here are some awesome and money saving Paleo non-grain tips to try put today!

On rare occasions, go for almond or coconut flours: Yes, these flours tend to be a bit pricey but as long as you use them on only the rarest of occasions, you should be good to go. One way to make the best of these flours without busting your budget is to use them in mousses and other very low-flour requirement recipes, allowing you to use just a little of these flours and still get your once in blue moon, Paleo dessert fix!

Learn to soak nuts and seeds, sprout them and turn them into your very own homemade flours: Almond and coconut flours can be expensive and can get repetitive if you only use the two, so instead, learn to make your own nut and seed flours.

Soaking your nuts and seeds before use will allow you to eliminate any unpleasant and potentially harmful enzyme inhibitors present in them. Additionally soaking allows us ot properly digest and utilize the nuts and seeds by helping the release of phytates, a potential risk in nuts and seeds (although occurring in much lower amounts within them than within grains) that could prevent the correct absorption of vital minerals.

How to soak your nuts and seeds:

1. Start with raw nuts or raw seeds.

2. Place the nuts or seeds in a large bowl (Ensure that it is large enough to handle any swelling in size that could occur) and pour filtered water over them until they are fully covered.
3. Allow them to soak in the bowl overnight.
4. Remove the water from the bowl, leaving the nuts or seeds behind.
5. **Your nuts or seeds are now cleared of excessive amounts of anti-nutrients and enzyme inhibitors, allowing you to either use them immediately or keep them in a closed container in the fridge for a couple of days.**

You may also choose to sprout your nuts and seeds. Sprouting is an entirely natural process that can ramp up levels of valuable nutrition within your nuts or seeds.

How to Sprout Your Nuts or Seeds:

1. Start with completely raw nuts or seeds that have already been soaked.
2. Place them on a large plate and arrange them so that they each have a little room between them.
3. Cover the nuts or seeds loosely with either a piece of unbleached muslin or a cheese cloth
4. Make sure that your rinse twice daily
5. When sprouting begins, it will be indicated by the appearance of a small white "tail-like" growth on the narrow side of the nuts or seeds
6. At this point you can use your nuts and seeds immediately or place in a sealed container in the fridge instead.

Top Tip: Use these soaked or sprouted nuts and seeds to make yourself a seriously delicious, nutrient rich and very inexpensive Paleo homemade granola. Dry your nuts and seeds thoroughly and toss them in the oven or dehydrator along with a good coating of raw, pure honey, a few drops of stevia, a pinch of nutmeg, cloves and cinnamon as well as bit of salt to season!

As soon as you get rid of the grains in your life, you will begin to feel and look more like you were always intended to, strong, healthy lean, happy and alert. You'll enjoy the anti-inflammatory benefits of having a glowing, youthful complexion, a light, agile and muscled body, an extra boost in your step, a continual natural energy and a quick thinking mind that won't let you down! No matter how much you adore donuts or live off of sugary cereals, trust me, nothing made of grains can ever taste as good as finally claiming victory over your health, weight gain and emotional as well as cognitive challenges, once and for all! You owe yourself a chance to see the amazing unfulfilled potential that grains have been keeping your from unleashing for many years. That's why I'm ending this chapter with a challenge: Try going absolutely grain free for 1 month. Within that time, do not consume any drink, food or snack with grains of any kind in it. Certainly, after the first addiction withdrawal pangs, you will find yourself looking and feeling lighter, healthier, more vibrant and vital than ever before. And I guarantee that once you've experienced your body and brain without grains, you'll get rid of this unhealthy strain for good!

www.ingramcontent.com/pod-product-compliance
Lightning Source LLC
Chambersburg PA
CBHW060324030426
42336CB00011B/1188